TODDLER DISCIPLINE

Written By

Jennifer Siegel

Table of Contents

INTRODUCTION

Thank you for purchasing this book!

Connection or secure attachment is one of the significant biological needs of humans. It is no surprise that children have a strong passion for their parents. Parents provide their needs for optimal development and survival. It is necessary to put your love into action, meet your child's needs, pay attention, respect his views, and instill loving guidance or discipline to establish a strong connection. Without secure attachment or when conditions are not satisfied, the outcomes are retardation of growth and occurrences of destructive behaviors.

During the toddler stage, your child wants independence but still afraid to be separated from you. He starts to realize that he has strong feelings, but does not know how to express or control them. Moreover, the child discovers that he has a power that can make others give him what he needs and will test it now and then. All these things are opportunities for parents to nurture their connection to their toddlers. The relationship is also the vital key that makes the child willing to follow the rules you set with willingness and cooperation.

Explain Yourself

At 24 months and up, toddlers are beginning to understand what is right and what is not. Unfortunately, it is also the stage where sharing is difficult for the child, not wanting to share your attention, time, or even toys. And what complicates the matter more is he begins to snatch everything he likes. The good news is that toddlers can comprehend the cause and effect and follow the simple instructions, so you can try saying, "We don't grab the toys of others" and give him his toys.

This is why you must explain to your child the reason behind your rule or instruction. It helps him see and decide which is the better option or behavior. Inform the child about your expectations, precisely the action you want him to demonstrate.

For example, you see your kid with a crayon and going closer to the wall. Refrain from yanking the crayon and yelling "no," instead hug him gently to divert his attention. You can also give him a piece of paper, explaining that coloring is nice, but it should not be done on the walls.

As much as possible, avoid telling him what not to do or stopping his attempt by saying, "no." According to child experts, toddlers who hear many "no" everyday display more deficient language skills. It also becomes ineffective when overused, prompting the kid to ignore it or shriek the minute he hears it from the parent.

Enjoy your reading!

Positive Parenting

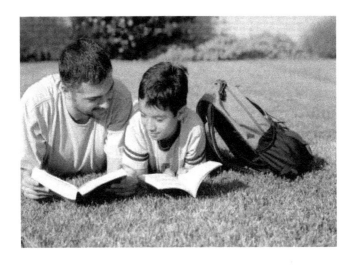

Positive parenting is defined as a style of parenting that emphasizes mutual respect. It is also referred to as gentle guidance, affectionate guidance, or loving guidance that places or keeps the child on the correct path. It uses positive discipline, instructions, and reinforcements geared at training the child to become a self-disciplined, responsible, and confident person. It involves teaching the child the who, where, when, what, and why of every situation. Its primary goal is to develop a deeply-committed, open, healthy, and strong relationship between the child and the parent.

It is an approach that helps children feel connected, connected, capable, and cooperative. It is not just about letting go of punishment or being permissive. Positive parenting is choosing to become actively involved in connecting and supporting their optimum growth and development. Generally speaking, positive parenting nurtures the child's self-esteem, sense of mastery, ability to interact, and belief in the future by living a productive, open, and healthy life.

Vital Elements Of Positive Parenting

- Imagine or understand the point of view of the child during challenging times.

- Provide consistent and age-appropriate rules, limits, and expectations.

- Respond with sensitivity and interest to the cues that the child displays.

- Recognize the child's abilities, strengths, and capabilities to learn and then celebrate them to reinforce the development.

- Enjoy moments of connection.

- Work to attain a balanced time for child needs and parental needs.

- Understand that missteps are part of rearing a child, and sometimes, parenting can be stressful.

- Learn how to regulate your behaviors and emotions before responding to your child.

- Seek support, help, and parenting information if necessary.

Studies show that the child's experiences in his first three years of life are influenced by the quality of caring that he receives from his parents—the efforts to nurture, support, and raise him set his path to success and happiness. His young brain is recording and assimilating everything, processing them as truth and proper. Your habits become new habits.

Effects of Positive Parenting

Positive parenting encourages children to respond to gentle guidance, improving their behavior, and developing self-discipline. In the absence of threats and punishments, children discover their strengths, power, and capabilities. It teaches children to accept their flaws or weaknesses and work to improve them.

It offers many benefits which include:

A. Maintaining quality parent-child relationship.

A fostering connection between you and your child is the foundation for developing good character traits, behavior, and confidence. Positive parenting is characterized by firm, loving guidance that builds a stronger connection and relationship. When you consider the long-term effects of positive parenting on your child, you know that you are on the right track.

The parental relationship is the most significant and influential connection that sets the bar for the child's cheerful disposition in life, success, and behavior. The strong bond fosters better decision-making, boosts self-esteem, encourage autonomy, and promote cooperation.

• Be involved. Enrich your relationship by connecting with your child using an age-appropriate approach. If your child is still a toddler, play with him, work on fun and creative projects, and teach him to read. If you have an adolescent child, challenge him in his favorite video game or sport. This technique will make him see you as an approachable parent.

• Emphasize on family time. A habit to eat dinner together or do something together during weekends. By establishing a regular family togetherness, you teach your child the importance of family as a unit.

• Set a one-on-one time for your child.

Spending quality time with your child is priceless. It helps you monitor his progress and development, making him feel your presence in every step of his journey as a person. Recognize his talents, strengths, and interests. Use the time to instill positive discipline by talking about situations that he considers problematic and finding ways to resolve the problems permanently. Build a meaningful and memorable bond by engaging in fun or educational activities.

• Get in touch with his academic and extracurricular activities. No matter how busy you are, making an effort to learn about his daily activities will make him feel loved and important. Ask about his friends at school, sit down with him when he is doing homework, help him check before the test, attend his school events, or invite his friends.

B. Taking responsibility for actions

Become the model of accountability by being humble and honest to admit that you are wrong. Teach him the importance of saying sorry and being responsible for his action or reactions over matters that affect relationships.

Before you can effectively teach your kid about taking responsibility for his actions, it is necessary to recognize and understand the "why" that triggers his behavior. There is a reason why he misbehaves, not just to get into trouble or annoy you. As a parent, you have to find it out in ways that will not offend, hurt, or embarrass him.

•Respond, but do not react. Avoid overreacting and take a deep breath. Do not force him to apologize or become accountable immediately. Give time for both of you to calm down.

•Make it safe for him to come forward. Once everyone is calm, let him approach you and explain his behavior or admit the truth. Another option is to approach him and talk about what happened. If he admits his wrongdoing and apologizes, you need to acknowledge the effort, discuss how it can be prevented in the future, and enforce his action's corresponding consequence.

• Stick to your rules and limits. No matter how pitiful his pleadings or how sweet he becomes after his misbehavior, it is essential to be consistent with your discipline strategy. Don't give in if you want to convince him that you are serious about the rules.

• Talk about action or behavior, not the person. Instead of pointing out your child's flaw, focus your attention on his behavior, and find the reason behind it. Let him voice out his sentiments, feelings, and thoughts. Empathize with his struggles, listen to what he is telling you, read between the lines, and work together to find an appropriate solution that will prevent the action's recurrence.

C. Being respectful to others

One of the goals of positive discipline and positive parenting is fostering mutual respect. Respect is a two-way process. If you want to raise a respectful child, it is essential to model the behavior. Home is the first place where he learns about this fundamental virtue, so you need to teach respect as early as possible.

• Lead by example. Kids are very impressionable. They naturally mimic the habits of people who are around them while growing up and look up to them as role models. Start teaching your child the value of respect, living a respectful, and leading a loving and kind life.

• Use respect as a tool for him to get what he likes. In the adult world, people who show affection are most likely to get what they want. Teach this to your child by only giving the something he wants when he is respectful. He will soon realize that it is a quicker and smarter way rather than throwing a fit.

• Encourage activities that require cooperation and sharing. One example that teaches these virtues is a board game. Every player needs to respect the time that other players take to consider their moves.

•Be patient. Patience is a manifestation of respect. To teach it effectively, you should not display impatience when you are dealing with him. If he observes that you are not practicing what you are telling him, he will not imbibe the true essence of patience.

D. Knowing the difference between right and wrong.

Recent studies revealed that 19-21 months old babies could understand the sense of fairness or the right from the wrong. The quality of care that children experience in the early months of his life lays the foundation of a positive parent-child relationship. The first five years of their lives are crucial periods of moral, social, and emotional development. Their understanding of justice and fairness expands as they grow.

At ages 0 to 1, the infant learns right from wrong through experience. He feels that something is wrong when he is wet or hungry. If he is adequately attended and nurtured, he feels good and right. By the time he is 1-year old, he can communicate his feelings through actions and preferences, initiate contact, imitate, and develop a deeper understanding of what is right to do and what is not.

At ages 1-3, the toddler learns to understand the concept of rules. He responds and stops his attempt if you tell him not to do something. However, sometimes, he cannot resist acting impulsively, like grabbing a toy from another child. At this period, he still cannot truly distinguish the right and wrong acts. The child relies on you or other pictures of authority to define them for him.

At ages 4-5, the preschooler child begins to develop his ideas of what is right and wrong based on what he sees and learns from the family. As his social exposure and interactions increase, the child's moral intelligence grows too. He becomes more aware of acceptable behavior and begins to develop a stronger sense of justice. At this stage, you need to be more vigilant and consistent with your reminders.

•Initiate discussions about ethical situations and encourage your child to talk about his feelings. It leads to the development of values and ethical behaviors that will guide him in his lifetime.

•Let him understand that people have different feelings and thoughts. This will develop his capacity to observe and respect other people's feelings, learning to respond with concern and care.

•Help your child understand his feelings. Make him realize that emotions are not wrong or right, but how he acts or reacts makes a big difference.

•Regularly discuss with your child your decisions or behaviors in the context of right and wrong.

E. Making good and wise decisions.

Decision making is a vital skill that your child needs to develop to become successful in all aspects of his life, especially when he becomes an adult. The choices and decisions he makes dictate the path and direction of his adult life. Thus, the importance of teaching your child how to make wise decisions.

It is necessary to teach him as early as possible because once he goes out to start interacting with the outside world, external influences will attempt to steal the decision-making from him. Most children who are good at decision making become victims because the popular culture easily sways them.

F. Being honest, trustworthy, and loyal.

Before you can effectively discipline your child, it is essential to affirm or reaffirm your connection by being honest with your feelings.

• If you want him to study, tell him how proud you are for the high score during the last examination.

• If you are nervous about how he runs across the parking lot without looking first on both sides, tell it to him.

When you impart your feelings, he is more likely to follow your wishes, creating a life-lasting pattern of making him anticipate or be concerned with others' feelings before acting.

Positive Communication

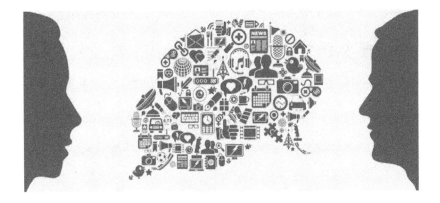

When my daughter wants to share information, she often asks, "Can I tell you something?" It's one of my favorite habits because I get to respond, "You can always tell me anything." Whether she's telling me about her joys and fears, how she's a part cheetah and part vampire, or plans for her birthday party, my intention is the same: to let her know that I am always there for her.

Communication is a top priority in our house. We tell our daughter we will always love her, no matter what. We tell her when we are getting frustrated. We talk about everything. I tell her she can ask me any question; I won't always have the answer, but she and I can find it together. All of this promotes a feeling of security and connection.

But this makes it sound easy. Real communication isn't always accessible or natural. It takes work and practice because what's easy is getting caught up in thoughts or distracted by automatic judgments or other things.

Intention And Connection

Our choices are a vital foundation for good communication. Setting the intention to care first and foremost, to be open to what the other person is sharing and experiencing, and to be curious but nonjudgmental allows for real listening and connecting. We often come into a conversation with a specific, narrow agenda or distracted by other things, which tends to close us to a real exchange.

As with any other skill, good communication takes practice. This doesn't mean rehearsing what you're going to say but practicing noticing your intentions as you begin a conversation and working to be present, mindfully, and judgmental. You can do this with your children and your partner, co-workers, friends, or other family members. Notice if you've decided how the conversation is going to go before you start. Inhale before you speak and, while the other person is saying, see if you can be open to what this person might offer (even if you disagree). Notice what it's like to be curious and care about connecting with this person, in whatever way is appropriate. The practice is vital because we are trying to build new habits, and when we are tired or stressed, we tend to fall back into our old, not always helpful patterns.

With positive parenting, we want to prioritize connection first and foremost. This isn't just about getting children to do something or having our say. How we say something often matters more than what we say. If we come to a conversation agitated, stressed, and distracted, our children will feel and feed off that and will be less likely to feel connected to us. If we are focused on being present with kindness and curiosity, they will feel heard.

Not every conversation needs to be an in-depth, life-changing discussion. You could have meaningful conversations when you pick the kids up from school or when you are asking them if they brushed their teeth. It's about choosing to connect first.

Listening

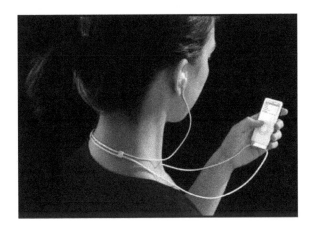

Just like us, children want to be heard. And although we want to be good listeners, life often gets in the way. Think about how often your child gets interrupted. It's probably a lot. When we interrupt them, we give them the message that what they have to say isn't necessary. Admittedly, your four-year-old's treatise on dinosaurs might not be the most scintillating thing you've heard. But again, this is about the long term. We inform them that we care, and their voices matter.

This isn't to say that you can never interrupt. If your child is anything like mine, you might have to interrupt; otherwise, you won't get a word in at all. We want to be clear about the intention to listen and be present for what they have to say.

Likewise, think about how many times we say things like, "You can't possibly be hungry; you just ate," or "Why are you so tired? You had a good night's sleep," or "But you love your gymnastics class." It's natural to react this way, but once we do so, we've not only closed ourselves off to hearing what's going on, but we might also be leading our children to doubt that we trust them, making it less likely that they will continue to be open and honest with us about how they are feeling.

To foster trust, build more connections, and promote our children's healthy development, it's essential to seek to understand their needs and their position. We need to listen openly and with the intention of closeness, without preparing a response in advance.

We just listen to what they say. It makes a more significant impact to be open to what they are feeling and going through and to let them know we care. When they say something that gets our blood boiling or makes us concerned, we have the opportunity to be aware of those reactions, to check our nervous systems, and then to communicate openly back to them: "I hear you saying that you want to ___. That makes me feel nervous. Can we talk about it some more?"

You might consider scheduling a monthly family meeting or event that lets everyone share openly. Conversations over the dishes are good, but it's useful to supplement them with time devoted to communicating. This also enables children to know there is always space for them to share. And yes, if you have older kids, this suggestion might engender serious eye-rolling, but that's mostly unavoidable at this point, so you might as well go for it anyway.

Talking

It is helpful to have specific techniques for communicating. Our approach in this book is based on nonviolent communication (also known as compassionate communication). Pioneered by Marshall Rosenberg, it's an approach that offers specific strategies to build on the innate human capacities for compassion and empathy.

Generally, it's more supportive of expressing what's going on in terms of what you see and how it makes you feel rather than what the other person is doing or automatic reactions. "You are so frustrating" can shut down the conversation a lot faster than "I feel very frustrated right now."

This approach follows four main components, which both the speaker and the empathic listener use.

1. Observations: saying/receiving what you see, feel, hear, remember, imagine as objectively and nonjudgmentally as possible

2. Feelings: saying/accepting what you are feeling, expressing emotions

3. Needs: sharing/receiving empathically what needs are not being met

4. Requests: offering/hearing concrete ideas that would help meet your needs

We can use the ubiquitous "clean your room" argument to illustrate what this might look like.

Scenario one:

After a stressful day, you see your child's room. It's filthy. You immediately get angry. This is the millionth time this has happened. You begin yelling, "I've asked you a million times to clean your room. It's disgusting! I don't remember you listening. Why can't you do what I ask for once?"

Now, imagine the child's reaction. Most of us can understand the parent's perspective, but these statements are full of judgments, blaming, and personal criticism. The child will likely feel attacked and possibly lash out in retaliation, leading to more arguing and less connection (and less room cleaning). This method of communication is more about punishment and autopilot than discipline and conscious response.

Scenario two:

After a stressful day, you see your child's room. It's filthy. You immediately get angry. This is the millionth time this has happened. You want to start yelling. You stop yourself and take a breath (or a more extended break) to decide how to deal with this situation before responding with: "I see there are clothes all over the floor and the bed isn't made. I'm feeling frustrated. I've asked you to clean it many times. It seems you don't respect the rules of the house that are important to me. Can you please clean everything up before dinner?"

You can imagine the child's reaction here, too. Besides looking at you like you've grown a second head because you're weird, this will make them pause. You aren't attacking or blaming. You are presenting the situation so that everyone can relate to it, and you're allowing them to respond.

How you apply this will vary widely depending on the situation and the age of your children. Yet even with a toddler, you can say, "I see dirty hands. That can lead to germs. Let's go wash our hands together."

And of course, nothing is magic. Communicating more effectively does not mean your child's room will stay clean, that they will listen, or that all yelling will cease. It's helpful to practice compassionate communication, but this is still a child's room (or curfew, or homework, or any of the other challenges we face) that we are talking about: They are rites of passage and aren't going away any time soon. But even if your house stays messy, you've opened up the path to tremendous respect, trust, and listening through more open, compassionate communication.

Conversation Traps

Most of us regularly fall into certain unhelpful traps in conversations. The goal here isn't to beat ourselves up about them but to do our best to see when we fall into these traps, forgive ourselves, and then choose an approach that promotes more give-and-take. Some common downsides:

•Blaming the other person or ourselves: Even if someone is at fault, we want to encourage taking responsibility rather than casting blame.

•Global judgments: It's better to stay specific than to make overarching statements about ourselves or others.

•Black-and-white statements: There's almost always an exception to the rule. "Always" and "never" reports cut off chances for growth and change and make others defensive.

•Unhelpful listening: This includes not listening at all but also rushing in to advise without being asked, offering pity rather than empathy, one-upping the other person with our own story, or when a conversation turns into an interrogation.

Other Helpful Communication Hints

Use do statements instead of don'ts: "Hold the cup with two hands" is a lot easier to follow than "Don't spill." It's tough for anyone to comply with a "don't" statement because it's not clear what should be done instead. To support our children better, it's best to use positively framed ideas.

Talking to them directly: Parents often talk to their partners or other adults about the children rather than talking to them. Part of empowering our children means trusting their (age-appropriate) maturity and responsibility. Understanding their level (for little ones) is crucial.

Use fewer words: Parents tend to over-explain and lecture when merely pointing something out is more effective. "I see dirty clothes on the floor" has more impact than "Your clothes are on the floor again. I've told you a hundred times that you have to pick up your clothes. You need to take more responsibility for yourself, et al."

Ask questions: Instead of lecturing, which they tune out anyway, get them involved. Ask your children, "How can we solve this?"

Behavior

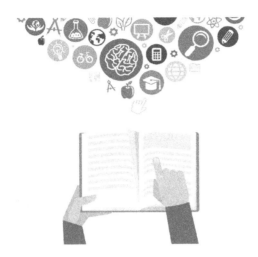

It's necessary for parents to bear in mind that kids are naturally good, and they have episodes of acting up due to specific reasons that they cannot voice out, especially when they are young and don't know how to process their emotions.

There are two factors behind your child's challenging behavior: the sense of not belonging (connection) and the sense of significance (contribution). When one or both basic needs are not satisfied, the children find a way to fulfill it, even if it requires adverse action. Dr. Dreikurs aptly put it by stating that "A misbehaving child is a discouraged child."

Calling the child as "bad" for doing something negative isn't healthy for their self-esteem. It usually starts when your kid continually misbehaves or throw tantrums, and you are exasperated. While trying to calm them, you lose control and label them as a "bad boy" or "bad girl" unintentionally. You can forgive yourself after that little slip and quote the famous cliché that you're just human, and humans make mistakes, but if you keep repeating it every time they do something wrong, it will be engraved in their mind and damage their self-worth.

Positive discipline aims to help parents learn to objectify the behavior and cut the "bad cycle." For example, instead of telling your child when they hit their younger sibling that "that's bad" or "you're such a bad boy," you may say, "it isn't okay to hit your brother when you are angry because they do not share their toy" and then let them understand the harm that might happen to their brother. When you objectify their behavior, you're teaching them the cause and effect. By directly addressing the "bad behavior" without using the term "bad," you're encouraging your child to make better choices and avoid hurting other people.

Show the child how to resolve the problem, instead of pointing out that what they did is wrong.

Redirecting your child's behavior requires more than saying, "Don't do that" or "No." It needs skills to teach them right from wrong using calm actions and words. For instance, you catch your child before they can hit their little brother, instead of saying "No hitting" or "Don't hit," tell them to "Ask their brother nicely if they want to borrow a toy." Other means to grab the toy, you're showing them that asking is more effective than hitting.

If they already hit their brother, it's a must to be creative with your response. One right way is enforcing a non-punitive time-out, which technically is about removing the child from the stimulus that triggers their behavior and allows them to calm down. You can cuddle them when they are agitated, let them play in their room, or ask them to sit with you and read a book. After their emotion subsides, start explaining (not lecturing) why their behavior is inappropriate. Please encourage your child to give other positive options that they believe will provide them with the result they want, without hurting anyone.

Be kind, yet firm when enforcing discipline. Show respect and empathy.

A child may insist that what they did was right, hence the importance of enforcing safety rules and consequences to prevent similar incidents in the future. Listen to their story as to why they did it and win half the battle by displaying empathy, but still impose the consequence of their action to learn from their mistakes. Kindness makes your child feel understood, lessening their resistance, and heightened emotions.

Look for the "why" behind this behavior, especially when you observe a pattern. Sometimes, hitting a sibling is a silent message that they are jealous of the attention you're giving to the younger child. Whatever the cause, resolve the issue early to make your child feels secure and loved. Get to the bottom reason of the problem.

Offer choices, whenever possible.

Giving your child positive choices works like magic when disciplining them. An example is when you're trying to make them sleep, and they still want to watch TV, instead of getting angry, provide choices. "Do you like to go to bed now or in ten minutes? Ten minutes? Okay, ten minutes and then off to bed."

This approach is a win-win solution because they get to pick the option that is okay with them, and you're offering choices that are advantageous to you. By not forcing them to do something and letting them choose, you prevent power struggle. You allow them to take charge and show autonomy within your parameters. To successfully use this technique, provide palatably, but limited choices. Eliminate options that are not acceptable to you and honor what they select.

Use mistakes as learning opportunities for your child.

Use every misbehaving episode as a chance to learn invaluable life lessons. Often, the child misbehaves to achieve what they want or when they are bored. For instance, they throw and break toys when they do not like them anymore. Instead of scolding them, use the opportunity to teach them the idea of giving them to their friends, or donating them. If they are bored, provide other exciting activities. This will teach them the concept of displacement or finding ways to be productive and prevent their properties. By empowering them with alternatives, they will be adept at making wise choices, even if you are not with them.

Prevent the repeat of misbehavior by changing the scene.

The famous adage still works – "Prevention is better than cure" in positive discipline. If you notice that your child keeps repeating an act, find ways to prevent it from recurring or resolve the problem.

One significant reason that you need to look into consideration is a transition. Most children do not like sudden changes, even in the ordinary routine. For instance, your child hates brushing their teeth in the morning and would do anything not to do it. Naturally, you will be frustrated because of the daily ordeal of resistance, which they show by crying, whining, screaming, hitting, or kicking.

What happens? It shows that they aren't resisting the act of brushing teeth; they are against the transition from sleep to a busy day because it overwhelms them. So, the next time your child repeats their tantrums over something, get to the leading cause and allows a transition time. For example, instead of rushing them to get dressed, set a timer that lets them do what they want, including getting ready. Ask him- "Do you need 20 or 30 minutes to get ready?" By letting them decide, they become in-charge of the allotted time but know that they need to show up dressed up before the time is up.

Be well-defined and stable with your expectancies and boundaries.

Children always find ways to push beyond the limits or find loopholes to satisfy their whims. They will attempt to test the limits to see your reaction or challenge you to know what will happen. So, it's necessary to talk to your child about the boundaries you set and the things you expect from them. Explain the corresponding consequences when they violate limits or house rules.

It is also essential to be consistent and follow through (do what you say) because it shows that you're serious about discipline. By being consistent, you're teaching them self-discipline, self-control, and other valuable lessons in life that will come in handy when they become an adult. Discipline requires a consistent application to be useful. Over time, they will recognize that their behavior and actions lead to consequences that they despise.

Use questions, state facts, or single-word reminders, instead of demanding or ordering them to comply.

When your baby grows into a toddler, you need to find language to make them comply and cooperate. Using respectful words is essential to make them obey you without saying "Stop" and "No." Connecting with your little child required breaking down communication barriers since they are still developing their speech skill.

It's much better to say, "Please look to your left and right before crossing the street," instead of ordering, "Don't cross the street without looking on your right and left." The word "Don't" serves as the modifier that confuses a little child. Say, for example, even if you cry out, "Don't jump in the puddle," your 2-year old kid still jump in and wonder why you're annoyed.

Treat and talk to them like an adult. Instead of ordering them, use positive phrasing, open questions, single-word reminders, or facts.

Use, "Shall we get up now?" instead of "Time to get up!"

"Shall we put these away, so nobody trips over them?" instead of yelling, "Put them away!"

"Your face is covered with chocolate! What shall we do about it?" instead of "Wipe your face."

"Light" instead of "Turn off the light after using the toilet."

"Kind words, please." instead of "Don't speak like that."

"Water is wasting," instead of "You are wasting water."

"We need to look after your little brother.", instead of "Don't hit the baby!"

How can we solve this problem?

Be generous with reasons, background information, facts, and explanations, so your child will better comprehend why they aren't allowed to do something or why they need to do it.

Involve them in problem-solving by working together as a team to find a mutually agreeable solution.

Children behave better on their free will when they see parents as allies. By giving your child a voice and the opportunity to be heard, they become more cooperative. Brainstorm solutions together and allow them to provide suggestions on matters that ensure safety and well-being.

Allow your kid to face natural consequences.

There are two types of consequences-natural and made-up. The latter are those that you make to suit your needs and propel them to comply. Some experts say that made-up consequences are punishments in disguise.

Categorically, made-up consequences come in forms of immediate effects, fair results, and logical development.

Immediate consequences help you teach the child to realize that their behavior is tied up with a result. An example is losing their phone privileges for a week when you find out that they are lying about getting their homework done.

Fair consequences are those that are reasonable and not overly harsh. If you ground them or prevent them from using electronics for one month, your kid would not think it's fair, and you are doing an injustice. They will fight the consequence every step of the way and try to defy it when you aren't around.

Logical consequences benefit children with specific behavior problems. An example is disallowing them to play with their toys if they refuse to put them back on the shelf. By linking the consequence with the problem, you let your child see that their choice directly results.

Natural consequences are part of natural growth. When you allow your kid to make mistakes and experience the natural results that arise from their misbehavior, you're showing them that inappropriate actions can lead them into trouble or face immediate consequences beyond your control.

For example, they touch the hot pot and get their hand burned. The pain is the natural consequence, teaching them not to do it again.

Self-Efficacy And Self-Confidence

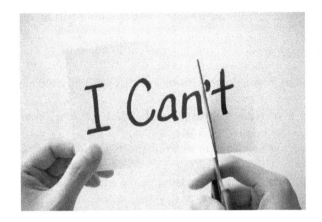

Self-Efficacy

Some people work hard and strive for success, whereas on the other side, people just let their life pass without any specific aims or perspectives. People tend only to try things; they will believe they will be successful. For example, you work at a store, and they ask you to create a spreadsheet on the monthly sales. In your entire life, you have never created a spreadsheet. It doesn't mean that you should refuse the objective given; instead, you should strive and learn the spreadsheet to make a monthly sales report. If a person thinks that he can accomplish a task, the person will have a higher self-efficacy. On the other side, if the person feels that he cannot achieve the given mission, his self-efficacy level is low.

Several factors influence Self-efficacy:

- Performance Accomplishments: It means that how successful you have been in your past related to a specific task. Suppose you have applied for a course to learn PowerPoint. If you had no difficulty understanding the time, you would feel more confident in performing a task in the future related to PowerPoint. This means that you will have higher efficacy for this type of study. On the other hand, if you had issues in learning the course, you will hesitate to work for that field. Therefore, your efficacy level will be lower in the related field to that course.

In the children's case, your child would be more confident if he had easily accomplished the task before. Or else, the child would fear to try to do the homework again as he doesn't have trust in his abilities. This means that the child lacks self-efficacy. Parents should always boost their children for trying new things, and they should make sure that the child is happily engaged in the work. The first impression of anything on a children's brain will remain forever.

- Vicarious Experiences: It means to observe someone very similar to you. You will keep and implement the things in your life. For example, if your co-worker is working hard on a project and is trying to produce a great outcome, you will try to act similarly. Your efficacy level will increase, and you will have a very similar result. However, on the other hand, if the co-worker is struggling with a project and finding it hard to produce a result, your efficacy level will drop. You will also find it hard in that project.

In the case of children, they tend to follow their parents or their siblings. Sometimes we see children following the activities of their friends or siblings. If a random child is active in building a castle at a beach, your child will also make a higher efficacy. This means that the child has boosted his effectiveness by vicarious experiences.

- Verbal Persuasion: This is very similar to encouraging someone for a particular task. For example, if someone encourages you by saying, "You can do this.", the efficacy level will increase. However, on the other hand, if someone discourages you by saying, "This is too much for you." the efficacy level will decrease, and you will find it hard to complete that task.

The children are susceptible to verbal persuasion. If you keep on discouraging your child, this will have a disastrous impact on the child's brain development and growth. The entire personality will be ruined. They won't be productive in any part of life, and they would be scared of implanting new things. Moreover, they will not get curious about new learning activities. The discouragement would have a significant impact on their brain. Therefore, it is recommended to boost your children's courage and potential by continuously motivating them and encouraging them. Most importantly, they would be more productive if they hair praise for their effort than their abilities.

- Physiological States: It depends on the emotional state, mood, anxiety level, et al. If you are healthy, your efficacy is higher. If you are feeling low or sick, your effectiveness is more inferior.

In the case of children, it is linked with their health. If the child is healthy and active, he will have greater efficacy than a child feeling sluggish and sick all the time. The parents should keep great care of their children's health. Make sure that the immune system of the children is fully active and healthy. A slight distraction can bring massive harm to your child. Apart from this, keep interacting with your children. This will help you understand their problems and make a stronger bond with them. Their physiological state will improve with your little attention.

Self-Confidence

It is the courage and ability to accept yourself or to believe in yourself. The definition is not sufficient itself, so let's give you an example. Suppose you are working in an organization, and you are a very hardworking employee. One day, your boss asks you to provide a presentation to the buyers. The buyers are essential for the organization, and the boss doesn't want to lose them. At this point, you have immense responsibility and pressure on your shoulders. Many of the people lose their skills, courage, abilities, and potential at this point. They lose their self-confidence and shiver with fear and anxiety. If you have self-confidence, you will have believed in yourself and your skills. You would have shown a more significant outcome than an average employee. Self-confidence provides the courage and ability to get your point of view approved. If you have self-confidence, you can achieve your goals.

Look around at those politicians; they dare to get their words approved in the assembly. From where do they get this potential and courage? It is all from self-confidence. To stand against the opposition, one must believe in oneself. If they don't believe in themselves, everyone will ignore their point of view. They will not be considered an essential part of the assembly. To be self-confident means you think the issues you are presenting and perusing people to follow it. Many of the great influencers, presenters, and speakers have self-confident. They know the way to keep their audience attracted to themselves. This is their skill, and they have trust in their mastery. For a more excellent example, refer to the motivational speakers. Look at the way they keep themselves attached to the audience. In no time, they create a bond with the viewers. Instead of fearing the people's reactions and views, they stand firm and deliver their thought with a great strategy. The strategy is nothing but self-confidence. Self-confidence is generated and build with experience.

The following factors influence self-confidence. The following factors are linked with the development of parent's self-confidence. The child learns from their parents, and the parents must develop self-confidence in themselves.

- Identify your negative thoughts: Your negative thinking creates a hindrance in your path to success. As we have learned in the belief system, the negative analysis is created by the conscious mind, and it harms the subconscious mind. Our self can control these negative thoughts. It just requires some motivation and uplifting. To boost and build your self-confidence, one must identify its negative thoughts and convert them into positive ones. Think more positive than negative; give complimentary analysis more space in your brain than negative reviews. The subconscious mind is like a warehouse, and filling it up with positivity will boost your self-confidence. Avoid unnecessary things that lower your self-confidence. Give time to yourself and mark things that disturb your peaceful mind. Filter them out, and you will observe the happiness in your life.

- Maintain a positive support network: If people keep on discouraging you, you will have low self-confidence. Your social pressure and fear will increase, and you will not interact much with the outer world. Let's take an example; you are a child whose parents keeps on discouraging their child by saying that the child is not capable and is weak. Even though the child is all good and perfect, he will feel sad and have lower self-confidence. This is just a small example related to motivation. If someone motivates you, you perform better. However, if someone continuously disturbs you and discourage you, the person will think negative of himself and will remain in depression. It is recommended to keep a positive support network. Stay in people that help you in your difficult time and stand beside you whenever you need any help. "A person is known by the company he keeps."

- Identify your talents and make a productive lifestyle: Keep yourself involved in your habits and interests. Permit yourself in taking pride in them. Express yourself through different hidden talents of yours. You will feel unique and accomplished. A greater probability of finding a compatible friend in your field of interest. Believe in yourself and start taking pride in yourself. For example, if a person loves singing and music, he will keep himself involved in his free time activities. He will have no time to think about the negativity around him. Interestingly, he can earn from his interests. This will make him more confident and will make him more relaxed in a hectic life. Moreover, accept the compliments gracefully. If you have a lower self-confidence level, you will find it hard to get a compliment from somebody. You will think that the person is either lying or mistaken.

- Stop comparing yourself with others: This is the biggest hindrance in the path to self-confidence. In this world, nobody is equal. Everyone has its potential, stamina, thinking, capabilities, strategies, et al. Don't make your life as your best friend's life. Think differently and make life as you desire than the desire of the people around you. Try to stand aside from the crowd as it requires self-confidence to be different.

- Learn from your mistakes: This is the essential tip in boosting your self-confidence. The ego destroys the personality of the people. Don't let your inner ego ruin your impression in others' eyes. If you work on your mistake, you will excel in your life. Don't lose hope by failing at one time. Keep on trying and trying until to succeed in your task.

How To Solve Conflicts

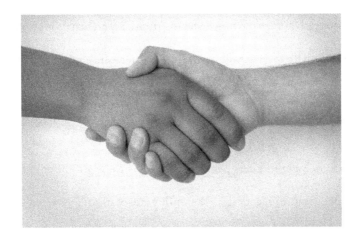

As your toddler increases in independence and begins to exert her will on the world around her, she will inevitably experience conflict. Conflicts may occur with siblings, other children, and adults—including yourself!

Helping your baby learn to manage conflict in safe and healthy ways is vital to his development. Many parents feel that toddlers aren't cognitively developed enough to learn how to solve disputes, instead opting to solve conflicts for their toddlers whenever possible. While there will be times when the safest or appropriate action is for you to take care of a problem from your position as caregiver, there will also be many times when conflicts are an opportunity for you to teach your toddler necessary skills in self-regulation, communication, and social interaction that will provide a solid foundation for more complex situations in the future.

The best way to help toddlers learn how to handle conflict is to allow them to experience it safely, with guidance and support when needed. When done effectively, taking advantage of these teaching moments to help your toddler learn how to get along with others will contribute to her sense of self, improve her ability to self-regulate, increase her social awareness, and help her develop empathy.

The first step in helping toddlers navigate conflict is to be good examples of how to use effective communication and conflict resolution strategies ourselves. Toddlers who see parents yell, argue, become rude or mean, call names, slam doors, etc. are more likely to do those things. Modeling healthy and productive strategies for conflict resolution helps toddlers to develop a healthier and more effective plan themselves.

However, modeling goes beyond simple behavior. It's also a good idea to model thought processes in the moments surrounding the conflict. For example, during a stressful encounter at the bank teller drive-through window, one mother looked in the rearview mirror to see her toddler looking at her with wide eyes. Chagrined, she realized that she'd been more than a little short with the teller.

Before the teller returned to the window, mom pulled out a quick think-aloud strategy: 'Boy, it makes me a little mad that this lady can't help me,' she said. 'But I should be kind so that we can picture out the problem together. I think I'll take a deep breath. Will you help me?' She and her toddler took a deep breath together, and when the teller returned, mom finished the transaction much more calmly. By using a think-aloud strategy, she was able to model positive thought processes that take place in real-world conflict resolution.

As adults, we are often able to resolve conflicts without much help from others. But what about toddlers? How much should we help them solve the conflict?

Toddlers, especially 3-year-olds, are quick to turn to mom to solve conflicts for them. Your response to these requests may range from complete intervention in the case of safety issues, to prompts and guidance as toddlers learn to handle conflict themselves, to be aware but hands-off as you let your little one try to solve the problem on his own.

As long as safety isn't an issue, a good rule of thumb is to let your toddler try to work it out on her own. Doing so will give her the experience needed to internalize successful conflict resolution strategies. However, as you move your toddler towards increased independence in handling conflict, you will still need to stay aware of the situation at hand and be ready to offer guidance in the skills, strategies, and coping mechanisms required to keep safe, respect others and reach her goals.

As you help your toddler learn to deal with conflict, keep the following tips and strategies in mind:

Take a break. Teach your child that sometimes, conflict can be made more accessible by taking a break to calm down. In the beginning, you can simply remove them from conflict situations that have escalated.

Tell them that they 'need a break to calm down' and can come back when they're ready. Before they go back to the situation, make sure they understand why they took a break—to calm down. Later, you can move on to asking them, 'do you need a break?' when emotions start to escalate, encouraging them to regulate their emotions with more independence. Eventually, they may even 'take a break' of their own accord.

Encourage 'I' statements. Teach older toddlers to express the problem from their point of view and to listen to the point of view of others. For example, 'I felt sad when you didn't want to color with me because I just wanted to color too. So I took your crayons to make you mad.' Learning to state and understand the problem will help your toddler understand where conflict has arisen from. It will also help him to become more aware of his reactions. When the problem is clearly stated, you can encourage your toddler to think about choices for dealing with the situation, whether it originated in himself or another.

Make apologies. Encouraging toddlers to apologize after a conflict has been resolved helps them learn to take responsibility for their actions. It can also help them to reset after some intense emotions. When your child is 1, they probably won't be making apologies of their own, although you can model this behavior for them. When they are 2, apologies may consist simply of a single word: 'sorry.' Once your toddler is three, you can usually start directing them towards more meaningful apologies that acknowledge what was done wrong and what will be done better next time.

Problem-solve. If your toddler comes to you asking for help with a conflict, you may want to encourage them to solve the problem themselves. Validate their feelings and ask open-ended questions to get them thinking about what they could do to resolve the conflict. For example, 'Wow, I understand that she took your toy. That sounds frustrating. How could we get it back? How could we find a way to share?' You might suggest compromise strategies or offer guidance, but try to let your toddler choose how to solve the problem. Afterward, praise them for figuring it out themselves.

Step back. Allow your little one to solve her conflicts whenever possible. Taking a step back will allow him to learn from experience. However, that doesn't mean that you aren't aware or active in keeping an eye on the situation. Be ready to offer guidance if needed, but try not to take over unless necessary.

Be safe. Not all conflicts are benign. Watch out for safety issues and intervene immediately if necessary. During the toddler years, you'll especially want to watch out for thrown objects, pushing, hitting, biting, etc. If emotions or behaviors escalate and become unsafe for anyone involved, you may need to remove your child from the interaction. Usually, you can stop things from reaching that point by being aware of the situation and intervening before it gets out of hand.

Acknowledge both sides. If your toddler and a sibling or another child come to you together for help resolving a conflict, don't take sides. Encourage each participant to share their feelings and come up with ideas for solving the problem. Even if one child is clearly in the wrong, make sure that both leave the interaction with their respect intact.

Consequences From Improper Training Of Your Toddlers

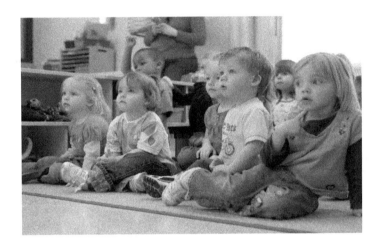

Parents must acknowledge that they are the ultimate reference materials for their children. To this end, the parenting method adopted in the training of the children has long-term and short-term effects on them. According to the 2011 report by the UK's Department of Education, it is understood that the conduct of children who had improper parental guidance is twice as worse as the average child. This was traced to inappropriate parenting done via physical punishment, verbal abuse, coercion, lack of interaction, and inadequate supervision.

1. Greater Vulnerability to Psychological Disorders: In light of a study published in a child development journal, it is understood that children who are directly or indirectly exposed to physical or verbal abuse in their early ages have a higher risk of having psychological disorders. In this study, there was no prevalence when the various psychological disorders are placed in comparison. However, these psychological disorders were all traced to factors in the early stage of children's development. It was found that the relationships with siblings in the family they come from or relationships with their parents had been injured. According to the Child Abuse & Neglect Journal, studies show that children who have been victims of abuse display post-traumatic stress disorder for a substantial period of their lifetime.

2. Defiance to Laws: In light of a research article published in the International Journal of Child, Youth, and Family Studies found that children who suffered parental negligence in their early days were more susceptible to being charged for juvenile delinquency. In this study, researchers were directed to investigate the connection between parental neglect and juvenile delinquency. However, some of the intellectual gaps identified in that study have been filled in other studies. One of these studies is the research published in Behavioral Sciences & the Law Journal. In that study, it was found that mothers who had once been charged with juvenile delinquency commonly

give birth to or nurture children with antisocial attitudes and tendencies to defy laws. According to the study, this was traced to parental abuse and negligence. In such cases, the problems of defiance to laws may be generational.

3. Depression: In the publication titled, "Parenting and Its Effects on Children: On Reading and Misreading Behavior Genetics," Professor Eleanor E. Maccoby of Stanford University explains that one of the causal factors of depression in children is parental adverse reactions toward their children. With these distinctive, credible articles reaching similar conclusions, it is hard to doubt that it is indeed true that factors such as overall support, verbal condemnation, physical punishment, and even depression of the parents are causal to the depression of a child.

4. Failure to Thrive: One of the implications of failure to thrive in toddlers is the retardation of mental growth, physical growth, and malnutrition. According to research submitted to the American Journal of Orthopsychiatry, it was learned that failure to thrive in toddlers is ultimately linked to parental negligence. Children who are victims of "failure to thrive" are found to have lacked good nutrition that is essential for healthy growth. This reduces its average growth rate. A publication in the journal Pediatrics

also traced the failure to thrive syndrome in toddlers to medical child abuse. It is found that parents who impose unnecessary medical treatments on their children make them vulnerable to the syndrome. In cases where your toddlers find it difficult to thrive, you need to check the medical procedures you have been exposing them to and the measure of care you show them.

5. Aggression: According to Rick Nauert's Psych Central article, "Negative Parenting Style Contributes to Child Aggression," the various research conducted by different specialists at the University of Minnesota all had similar conclusions; toddlers who were aggressive and quick to anger all had low interactions with their mothers. The decision was that one of the effects of bad parenting to toddlers is an aggression on the part of the children. The mothers studied treated their children aggressively, were verbally hurtful, and rebellious towards their children. The more negative parenting, the greater the child's aggression to colleagues will be. This created a certain level of hostility between mothers and toddlers. However, more research is now invested in knowing whether or not the relationship of the toddlers' fathers with their mothers influences the bad conduct of the mothers towards their children.

6. Poor Academic Performance: One of the consequences of parental neglect is the gross reduction in the toddlers' academic performance. This view is credited to a study conducted and published in the Child Abuse and Neglect Journal. The study concludes that when parents have minimal interactions with their children, it impairs the children's' learning ability compared to their peers. The children also lack social relationships. Further research shows that neglect is no less disastrous than physical abuse in terms of the toddlers' academic performance.

According to another study in the journal Demography, children whose parents always relocate or migrate also tend to poor performance in school. The truth is constant relocation is usually a factor that is above the power of the parents. Nonetheless, it may have detrimental consequences on the child's educational growth.

In terms of children's' mathematical performance, research has shown that the parents' mathematical interest can determine whether or not the child will be good at it. According to Melissa E. Libertus, an Associate Professor at the University of Pittsburgh, the connection is said to be either environmental or hereditary. In this light, parents that are easily provoked at their child's academic performance in mathematics should know it might have ecological or genetic causes.

Having seen some of the behavioral, cognitive, and social consequences of improper parenting, it is time you are introduced to a grand principle for training your toddlers.

Friends & Siblings

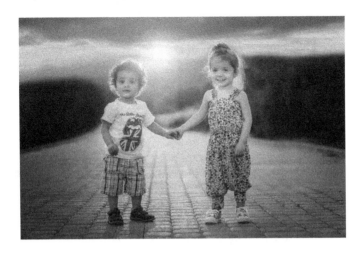

Can small children be friends? They can but in their way. That means you should be prepared to see one bite the other, take the toy without asking. These are things of the age that need to be understood. In the range of 1 to 3 years, the child is still selfish, and the question of the possession of objects is very present. Therefore, it is common for them to take a toy from the other's hand and walk.

The little ones are in the famous oral phase, in which they use the mouth as a means of discovering the world. As long as they do not know how to talk, they end up sometimes hitting for no reason, to get what they want. Of course, if aggressive behavior is too frequent and intense, it requires parental attention. It is unnecessary to deprive the one who was caught up in the other's life but to ensure that it happens in the most secure way possible, supervising and separating in case of aggression.

Not infrequently, a more passive child becomes friends with a bossy one. The experts consulted say that the leaderships of the group begin to dawn with 4 or 5 years. When this happens, others become his followers - and make no mistake about their little age: the leader realizes the strength his opinion has over others.

When the teacher identifies this in school, he should use strategies and jokes to dilute this configuration so that roles are reversed in some situations: followers become leaders, and the leader becomes a follower - this can also be done at home by parents. If conflicts arise from the relationship between a leader and a follower, it is recommended that each child should orally expose the other to how he felt and what he did not like. They should listen and try to resolve the situation with each other.

Shy Children

More introverted and shy children may have difficulty making friends. In such cases, parents may approach a class in the building's playground, for example, and introduce the child, asking if he can play with them. So, next time, he will already have a reference on how to act. You can also invite classmates to attend your home. That way, they will have what to talk about in the room, plus memories of fun times together.

But if the child is never called to any party and seems to be always isolated, the ideal is to do a job with the school to detect why this happens. You can also enroll your child in extracurricular theatre or sports classes that help decrease inhibition. Just do not press it.

If your child is amiable and makes friends quickly, rest easy. Just be aware of whether your child is not acting that way to get attention and can do a little more work with a classroom concentration. Point it out that there is time for everything.

Friends – Siblings

Who said siblings could not be good friends? In these cases, one only needs attention if the youngest becomes a" shadow "of the brother and ends up having no personality. Well, then, talk about the importance of having your attitudes.

There are also cases where siblings have no affinity. Parents should be aware of the context in which the lack of friendship happens and their expectations of that relationship. In general, siblings will be friends but often go through situations of jealousy and competition. They may also have different interests, which seems like a lack of friendship, but is related to gender and age. Parents need to look at how they relate to the family (mother, father, and siblings) to identify whether they have a strong or superficial bond because the child perceives and tends to have similar behaviors.

Leaving

If the parents look back, they'll remember that some of their friends walked away for a while and then returned. You have to stay calm and keep in mind that this is a process of building the child's bond. Another feeling that can arise in such a situation is jealousy. When there is some dependence on friendship, attention is needed. If we identify something negative, that does not benefit both parties. It is necessary to stimulate new friends. The adult should show that the child can discover affinities with several children.

Outside The Party

This will happen sooner or later, either for financial reasons (it's expensive to invite all the students) or affinity. In these situations, the adult needs to be prepared to face the child and parent's frustration. Parents must accept that it is not the end of the world and explain that some people identify more with each other than others.

The opportunity is ideal for sitting with the child and asking why he thought he was so close to the birthday boy. Sometimes he thinks he's friends with the other, but he's not reciprocated. It is essential to have this understanding that some people give the impression that they are our friends, but they are not.

Colorful Friendship

From the age of 4, children begin to perceive each other better, start comparisons, and have a more excellent perception of their own body. It is common for situations to arise from one wanting to kiss and embrace the other. Some even talk about dating. This is mostly a reflection of what they see daily in the media, that is, an imitation of behavior. When faced with such issues, parents should teach the child that he can express affection in various ways - with words, drawings, and jokes together - and to say that he should not kiss another person on the mouth.

My son never wants to leave his friend's house. What to do?

Parents should keep in mind that no matter how friendly they may be, there is no way to force children's bonds. The identity that made them be friends does not necessarily happen among their children. And adults should be prepared even to get upset. It would be better to avoid contact between children, especially when there are no others to interact separately. Prefer to date only with adult friends.

The Friend Is a Terror

You will meet those friends who are a "terror": they make a mess, they mess around the house, they speak profanity ... The desire to criticize the colleague can be enormous. If it is to your child that the message must be given, explain that there are several ways to behave and that the way the other acts do not please you, pointing out how the line has been crossed. The same must be done with swearing. In general, small children do not know what they mean, but if they realize that it causes anxiety in their parents, they can repeat it to manipulate them, just like the tantrum. Therefore, be very calm in explaining that this is not acceptable to say.

Away From Home

Generally, it is at about four years that the child starts to go to friends' houses and, from 5, can be prepared to sleep outside the home. Knowing the routine and habits of other families is positive, as it broadens the worldview. However, the child will inevitably make comparisons and question aspects such as "in so-and-so's house, I could stay up late. It is an excellent chance to teach your child that each family has its own rules that are not better or worse, just different.

It can happen the opposite; also: your son sleeps there and discovers that he does not identify with the family (schedule, food, fear of a pet). Heed what he has to share and do not force him back. One option to keep the friendship is to take walks with the colleague elsewhere or let your child visit you for short periods.

My Idol

It is common for children to choose a friend as an idol for a while and want to have the same clothes and toys or repeat their attitudes. Over time, they realize that they do not have to copy the colleague to have their friendship and stop it.

But it is good to be alert when this behavior is exaggerated, asking, for example, why the child wants an object or is doing it. Explain that friendship does not depend on it. If things got worse, ask help from a psychologist. At the other end, the "copied" child can tell his friend, "Be yourself."

Emotionally Intelligent Parenting

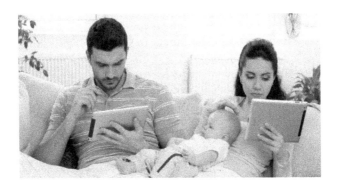

Emotional intelligence is one of the essential skills you need so you can live harmoniously with others. It allows you to get a grip on your impulses and keep a clear head when dealing with conflict. It gives the skills needed to maintain healthy relationships with the people around you. Keeping a tight grip on impulses is crucial when you are raising a child because the most harmful expressions of anger are those that happen instinctively. These include name-calling and spanking an unruly child in the spur of a moment.

Benefits of Emotional Intelligence

Impulse control

Even with a full understanding of your parenting style, you will be hard-pressed to continue acting in a levelheaded way when you are fuming at your child. A person with a high level of emotional control will understand the need to keep their head in charged moments to avoid hurting others. This is what emotional intelligence allows you to become. The higher your level of personal control, the better the power you will have over your impulses. This means that you will still have the presence of mind to take a moment to gather your wits before you start talking or lashing out when you are angry.

Dealing with crises

Emotional intelligence entails learning how to deal with problems in a sober manner. The ability to do this means that you never have to lose your head when there is a problem because you are confident in your ability to solve it. Feelings of helplessness play a massive part in parental anger, mostly because you are responsible for so much more than your child's needs. After all, the things you do to your child will affect their lives for years to come. The problem-solving technique of thinking about challenges helps to deal with anger because it gives you something to think about and will ultimately give you the solutions you need.

The most effective problem-solving technique entails;

1. First, seek to understand the exact nature of the problem. Sometimes our fears magnify small issues and make them appear more significant than they are. Define the issue in a statement, then twice more using different words. This allows you to determine what is essential in a situation.

2. Come up with a list of solutions to the problem. Brainstorm as many answers as possible without dismissing any one of them for the time being. Write down these ideas if you are afraid that you might forget them.

3. Go through the different solutions one by one and eliminate those that are non-workable. Narrow down the list of possible solutions until you have the best three.

4. Put the most promising solution to practical use and evaluate how effective it is. If it does not work, tweak a few things and then try out the next solution on your list.

5. Evaluate the whole situation and picture out if you are better off for it. For you to consider a problem solved, the case should improve significantly and visibly.

Anger and You

As a parent, you will get a lot of advice from friends and family to raise your child. Some of this advice may work, but most of it will probably not apply to your situation. Even worse, following some well-meaning advice often makes it even harder for you to execute your parenting duties. This is because you make the mistake of thinking that all parents deal with problems the same way. In truth, parenting styles vary and can be as unique as our different personalities. It is just the same way that children have other characters and present problems in unique ways.

Emotional Intelligence for Your Child

Emotional intelligence is not just a technique that a parent might use to manage their parental anger. It gives anyone who has mastered it the ability to express their emotions transparently and efficiently. It also allows for the mastery of emotional self-control, which means that you can picture out what you ought to say in front of people and those you should hold back. Children usually have none of these skills, and unless you teach your child to express themselves adequately from a young age, they might never master these skills.

Emotional intelligence allows a child to solve problems creatively and put up with others' emotions, especially when these emotions are negative. When you teach your child emotional intelligence, you teach him or her that feelings serve to make us know what we want. This way, a child learns to appreciate his or her feelings and respect other people's emotions. The most important aspect of teaching emotional intelligence is training your child on the practical strategies of dealing with negative emotions.

Parents deal with their children's negative emotions through one of the four methods: dismissing, disapproving, acceptance, and emotional coaching. Dismissive parents put little stock into their child's feelings and try to get rid of them as soon as possible. In a dismissive parent's point of view, a child needs only experience joy. Whenever they display a different emotion, a dismissive parent will use any distraction available to entertain the child back into happiness.

Disapproving parents rarely take the time to appreciate their child's feelings. At the first sign of negative feelings, they do everything possible to quash it by punishing the child. Punishments will often grow harsher as the child's unexpressed emotions grow more robust, and their expression more frequent.

Acceptance is pretty much how permissive parents deal with their children's negative emotions. They accept anything the child does without questioning or seeking to find the cause or possible solution. These parents are also called laissez-faire because they do not teach problem-solving or put any limitation of a child's expressions of negative emotions.

Finally, we have the personal coaching strategy of dealing with your child's emotions. This strategy views every expression of feelings as a teachable moment, and emotional coaching parents will usually take moments of a personal name to connect with their child. By pointing out how doing something can be bad for the child and other people, you empower them to rise above it and learn how to express themselves better.

Emotional Coaching

Take away from this book and it should be that your child's emotions are essential. This includes the feelings that follow your actions after your child has done something wrong. Children make the most meaningful choices when their emotions are raw.

You must be careful to ensure that these choices are the right ones for your son or daughter.

The five steps for emotional coaching

1. Notice your child's emotions. You must keep observing and reading into your child's actions and words. The best way of coaching your child to manage his or her feelings is to acknowledge them before expressing them. This gives you the time to picture out how best to handle when your child finally expresses the feelings.

2. Take the opportunity to strengthen the connection you have with your child. Find the best possible way of addressing your child's feelings and go with the most fun and pleasurable way of doing it.

3. Validate your child's feelings. No feeling can ever be wrong because all emotions are meant to show us what we need. Try to relate by actually putting yourself in your child's shoes. If you can connect with something from your own life, that might deepen the connection.

4. Clarify what the emotions indicate. As the parent, you are supposed to bring clarity to your child's confusion. It would help if you labeled the feelings your child is going through.

5. Guide your child to solve the problem at hand. The problem-solving step of dealing with negative emotions is crucial for building character. If you handle everything for your child, you risk making them too reliant on

your protection to manage their problems. Focus on teaching the skills of problem-solving and giving clues rather than providing solutions.

How To Replace Punishment With Positive Parenting?

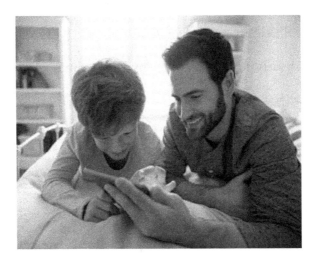

A positive approach to parenthood implies an understanding of the child and his or her behavior, paying attention to how the child feels. What does that mean practically? Seeing what is behind a child, 'child's action means seeing the real cause, understanding it, and offering the child an alternate solution to malicious behavior.

Adults mostly only see the "final product" – the unwanted behavior they want to correct, or a real cause. Suppose they want the child to learn something, and that isn't working. In that case, it is up to adults to explain to the child the consequences of his malicious behavior: natural effects ("You are cold because you do not want to wear a sweater.") and logical consequences ("We are late for the birthday party because you wanted to play even though the clock was ringing and telling us it was time to go.").

Positive parenting requires a calm tone of voice with an agreement and an explanation of what is acceptable and what is not and what will happen if the child does not adhere to the contract. Positive parenting creates a space for learning without guilt, shame, and the fear of punishment.

Children learn by making a series of efforts and mistakes. The whole process of a child's upbringing and learning is a series of attempts and errors until they master some skills. The role of the parents in this process is to provide direction and leadership. You must be a teacher to your children first of all, but a patient one.

Parenting is difficult and requires the patience to repeat the same thing hundreds of times. Being a child is also tricky because it requires strength and persistence to repeat the same thing hundreds of times until it is learned. This process cannot be accelerated, skipped, or eliminated. The least a parent can do is to change their perspective and accept that some things are slow and annoying and have to be repeated many times. Some parents have days when they feel discouraged because they have to repeat the same thing day after day. But that is also a significant part of parenthood.

One of the essential things in your child's learning process is learning how to live in the society in which he or she is growing up and learning the rules to function in that society. Kids have to know when it is proper and better for them to limit their autonomy and self-expression, and they have to know that they can do it. Then, they have to learn how to tolerate frustration and handle frustration and to be consistent despite it.

Without adequate limits in their environment, children feel agitated and unmanaged. Boundaries can be expressed as criticism and cause embarrassment, or they can be uttered in a reliable way - full of respect. Contemplate and speak the same way to your child. Do you respond better to vigorous criticism or respect, regard, and support? It's the same with your child.

If we allow them to, children will try to solve the problems they face in their development and upbringing. Parents often begin to scold or criticize the child, not expecting them to attempt to solve the problem. If the parents were more patient, they would be surprised how much their children can make conclusions and solve the problems they face.

Being heard is therapeutically potent and allows us to think about things clearly and find a solution. The same goes for children. Sometimes it's enough to listen to a child when they talk about their problems because they often come up with solutions that resolve the issues.

Fear and control are useful in the short term. Still, a child can become either completely blocked in his development or can begin to provide resistance to parental pressure through defiance and rebellion. Depending on the type of interaction a child has with their parents, the child forms a picture of himself and a sense of self-reliance in his roles in life. A blocked, non-progressing child has a lesser perception of his value, leading to isolation or it's opposite: aggressive and rebellious behavior.

Children should understand the importance of thoughts and emotions, not just behavior because it will enable them to function better in relationships with other people and deal better with problems. That is why adequate control of their emotions is an important skill, and one of parenting's most essential goals.

The words of parents and their assessments of a child are a mirror for that child. Children will see what their parents exhibit. That then becomes their picture of themselves, and they live with that. That is why it is essential to be specific and accurate with criticism. Criticism should be expressed with body language, which expresses regret rather than disapproval toward the child. The child will internalize a parental look full of condemnation and criticism, and we want to love and accept our children. This strong support for them will be the seed and the core of their happy life and success.

However, you should 't shouldn't give your child unlimited freedom; you do need to discipline them, of course. But how? Disciplinary measures respond to the child and his abilities and support the child in developing self-discipline. Discipline aims to target children, recognizing individual values, and building positive relationships positively. Positive discipline empowers children's faith in themselves and their ability to behave appropriately.

Discipline is training and orientation that helps children develop limits, self-control, efficiency, self-sufficiency, and positive social behavior. Discipline is often misunderstood as punishment, especially by those who apply strict punishment to make changes to children's behavior. Discipline not tantamount as punishment.

Instead of punishment, children need to be provided with support in the development of self-discipline. Positive discipline shows adults as pictures with authority that children allow developing strategies to control their behavior according to their age. Parents should take e a positive approach to discipline, developing positive alternatives to punishment.

Education is based on establishing and building relationships with your child, and the basis of each connection is acceptance, respect, and established boundaries. Setting the boundaries during your child's education is equally important as understanding, love, and support. In this way, children learn to be responsible for what is happening to them, and they are helped to learn self-regulation of their feelings and behaviors, gain self-confidence, and feel the confidence and trust of their parents.

Children know what is right and what is not. This is the knowledge that they adopt, and their parents are the ones who assist most in this. It's a formidable job, and children need the support of adults during this process. Parents need to learn how to stay patient and calm and help their child to learn in the best way possible.

Tips and Solutions for Peaceful and Positive Parenting

1. Speak in a calm voice - Rather than shout, talk with your child. This will help you to understand how kids need to feel a bit more of your patience. The way you react always influences the way the child behaves. Use positive parenting because it is vital for a healthy relationship between you and your child.

2. Give yourself a break - Patience is time-consuming. Sometimes it's hard to understand why your child behaves in a certain way and what you can do to help them. Patience is difficult when you have no time, and your child wants something from you. Patience is the power of understanding your child.

3. Try to understand your child - Understanding is the foundation of positive parenting and influences communication and respect. It is effortless to lose patience with a child you do not understand. Your toddler will always be a little nervous, tearful, angry, or just loud and not listening. However, you're a parent with unconditional love. If you ever try to talk to your child based on this unconditional love, you will surely understand him better and become more patient.

4. Let your child be independent - If you want to practice patience, put it to work in situations where you want your child to take on tasks for himself. Stop and allow the child to finish things. This is how the child will enjoy independence, and you, at the same time, will learn to be more patient.

5. Find the fastest way to calm yourself down - This is one of the most important things to learn about patience. Ways that can help you—for example, deep breathing. You can also count to 10, bake a cake, or something like that. You know what you can do to bring about quick relaxation.

The Power OF Empathy

Being an empathetic parent is the best gift a parent can give to their child. Your empathy for your child will let them understand that you actually 'get them.' Just like adults need someone to show confidence in them and acknowledge their feelings, so do young kids, especially toddlers. We need an understanding shoulder to lean on and cope with our time of distress. That shoulder will only be supported when the person understands where we are coming from and the reason for our present situation.

Toddlers are no different. They need us, parents, to be those understanding shoulders for them. We can become such strong support for them only by showing empathy. It is essential for kids that we understand them and their needs. For toddlers, their emotional needs and their feelings are of paramount importance. For us, a crying, whining, screaming, thrashing child might be just that, a child behaving undesirably. More so when according to us, they are doing so for no real reason and 'nothing.' But for them, it is hugely important. How many times have we encountered parents who defend their ignorance of their child's needs by saying it was 'nothing'? For us, it indeed might be nothing, but to them, it is as essential as the world.

Being empathetic toward your child gives you the space to see the world through their eyes. It makes space for your feelings without any judgment. Empathy is the great affirmation that toddlers need that tells them, "I understand how you are feeling. It's alright. Your feelings matter to me."

Empathy lets your child feel connected to you. It gives them a sense of belonging and security. They will be more at ease, knowing you are someone who understands them. This will bring more confidence in your relationship with your child. Children who have empathetic parents are more comfortable to "manage" and workaround. They live with the knowledge that they have support to fall back on bad days. If the parent is always critical and lacks empathy, the child will retreat within themselves. Such parents may be unable to foster a relationship based on trust and confidence with their kids. Such children will build resentment toward parents as time goes by. Empathy gives them the validation their feelings need.

Their mistakes are welcoming the very first step to validation. You are not accepting their behavior, instead of embracing that they are humans and will make mistakes just like you do. We are taught that mistakes are wrong from our early childhood, and the ones committing errors are wrong. We are taught that making an error is akin to failure. Children are innocent. They aren't bad, and they are pure. But when we are not welcoming of their mistakes, we are saying the exact opposite to them. When you are accusatory in your approach, kids resort to hiding and covering up their mistakes because they fear you. Hiding mistakes can never be a good idea, as one lie would need a hundred more to hide it. This is not a good trait to encourage in your child. When you hide wrongdoing, you can neither rectify it nor learn from it to avoid it in the future. Instead, be welcoming of their mistakes, guiding them gently to correct them with empathy. This is what validation gives them; a chance to get back up from their failures, learn from them and try not to repeat them.

Validation Versus Acceptance

Many parents confuse validating their child's behavior with accepting their behavior as correct. These aren't the same. The proof is to affirm the feelings of your child as something worth taking note of. You give their emotions the respect they deserve without brushing them off as inconsequential and meaningless. One of the biggest criticisms of empathy theory is that it encourages the child to feel confident about their mistakes and urges them to continue their bad behavior. This also isn't true.

Validation is not equal to condoning bad behavior. You are validating the way your child feels but not the way your child behaves. While you are empathetic toward your child by telling them how you understand their feelings and why they are angry or upset, you also firmly establish how you do not support or condone their bad behavior. See the following as an example.

A three-year-old is upset that her older brother has finished her orange juice. They both get into an argument, and she throws the empty juice carton at her brother, who ducks, and the open box lands on the side table, holding crockery, breaking a glass quarter plate and smashing it to pieces on the floor. Their quarrel and argument have resulted in a broken plate and the danger of strewn glass pieces all over the kitchen floor. Any caregiver would be angry. She was in the right by being upset, but was the ensuing argument and throwing things appropriately? How must the parent react? How would you react?

What the child needs here is for us to understand that firstly she is simply three years old. Just two years older from being a no-idea-what' s-happening infant. Only one year older from being able to talk. That is still a very young age for us to be taking them to the task. So what do we do? What that child needs are a hug and a rub on the back that tells them you understand. If it is a sensitive child, they would be crying even before you look at them. A more authoritarian child is bound to melt into your arms and call when you give that hug. Why is this so? Because at this tender age, kids are too innocent of fostering any real hate or negativity. Their guilt will bring those tears on. They are too overwhelmed by the loss of their juice and then the loss of their own emotions. You would only be hurting them more by scolding or yelling at them.

Once they have calmed down, the crying has subsided, and they can look at you without being uncomfortable; now is the time to tell them it was wrong gently. By this time, they know that already. But you have to lay down the rules when your child is calm and in a receptive enough state to listen and acknowledge what you are saying.

"I know you were upset. You were angry; your brother drank your juice. But, dearest, what just happened wasn't fine. You mustn't throw things at each other. We talk about and solve our problems. We do not throw things at each other. This could have seriously hurt someone."

This much is enough to let the message sink in. But this message will only get in their minds when you have held them and rubbed their backs, giving them that much-needed hug. That simple, empathetic gesture broke the barrier between the parent and the child. It is what made the child more accepting of their follies and the given advice. Of course, you mustn't forget the older brother or his part in this whole scenario, but for now, our concentration was the vulnerable little girl of three.

Validation is like saying I get how you are feeling. I'm afraid I have to disagree with what you have done, but I understand why you have done it. You can and must set behavioral limits while being empathetic at the same time.

Strategies on How to Empathize With Your Toddler

If you are looking to be empathetic to your child's feelings, there are a few things to keep in mind to convey the right message of understanding effectively.

- Bring yourself to their level. Either bend down or kneel so that you both are at the same level.

- Look your child in the eye and truly listen to them. Put away any phones or electronics, or any other chore that you might be doing, to give them your undivided attention.

- Reflect and repeat what they say. It is always a good thing to repeat what they tell you back to them. Doing this accomplishes two things. It means them you have understood what they are saying and opens for them a chance to correct you if you have misunderstood them.

- Describe how they look and give them words to help them tell you how they feel. For example, you may say, "You are pounding the table with your fists; you look angry!"

- Ask them appropriate questions, so you know you understand them correctly and validate their feelings and not the feelings you have chosen for them. For example, you might say something like, "You look sad, are you sad?" And then you let them agree or disagree.

- While being empathetic, do not criticize, judge, or try to solve their problems. Doing this would only defeat the purpose of being compassionate in the first place.

- Do not tell them, "You are feeling sad, so this is what you need..."

- Do not tell them, "Stop crying. If you go on crying, everyone will think you are a cry baby."

- Do not tell them, "You are always upset at the table during dinner."

Validating your child's feelings is just as important as teaching them manners and ethics. For toddler years, this is even more important as at this tender age, they are unaware of the complex emotions a human being is capable of feeling, and all that they undergo is bound to be overwhelming for an innocent mind. This age needs the most amount of validation and empathy to help the child learn the range of their own emotions and handle them.

Have a Meaningful Talk

Sometimes all you need is to sit and talk. Make it a point to have at least one meaningful conversation with your child every day. What you could do is have such a discussion at bedtime with your child. Before or after storytime, you could sit with your child and talk about your day. Then ask them about theirs and listen. It is remarkable how much a child is willing to share when you are ready to listen. Ensure that you end your conversation on a happy note that leaves your child smiling. Be it a joke, a funny story, a funny incident from your day at the office, or anything else, let the last memory of you be a happy one for your child as they drift off to sleep.

Having such sharing sessions is a step toward empathy. It will help you strengthen your relationship with your child and enrich the trust factor between you both. This is a valuable asset to have in your relationship as a parent as your child grows. With time, as your child grows and starts school, this same session will come in handy. Your child will be more forthcoming and trusting of you to share their day with you every day. This ease of conversation is what any parent desires, and you can have it too through a little empathy.

Teaching Your Child To Problem Solve And Be More Independent

There were so many times I have wanted to fix all my sons' problems. But I knew that I couldn't because I would only be holding them back instead of helping them. I want them to depend on me, come to me, and ask me anything. This is one of the biggest reasons I, like you, want to jump up and do absolutely everything I can for my children. As you do, I also know how this can keep them from going out in the world with confidence and learning from their mistakes. After all, making mistakes is one of the most significant ways we learn, grow, solve problems, and become more independent.

I understand when you struggle to take a step back and watch your child try to picture a new toy. I know how hard this is because it pains us emotionally to see our children struggle. However, I also know the thrill you and your child feel when they can overcome an obstacle. We often have tears in our eyes as we tell our child, "Good job! I am so proud of you!" I know I teared up when I've watched my children succeed. It's what we dream about as parents, even the little successes.

Tips on Teaching Your Children How to Problem-Solve

To do our best for our children, we often focus on the various information we receive from other parents. Therefore, I will share tips with you about how you can help your child learn problem-solving skills at any age.

Give Your Child an Obstacle

Giving your child a roadblock sounds like the opposite of what you want to do. However, think of it this way – if you can place an obstacle in front of your child, you can strategically. This means you can think about your child's problem-solving skills and make sure there is a solution for them to picture out. This will help them build their confidence when it comes to solving problems and allow you to see them thrive.

Don't Hover Over Your Child

I know we all want to do this. It's hard to see our babies grow up – actually, we always consider them our baby. But if you want the help, your child succeeds, you will know when you need to back away and let them take care of the situation themselves. For instance, your child comes home from school and tells you that another child pushed them. You look at your child and, while you want to go to your child's defense, you take a deep breath and ask them what they did. Your child responds, "I told them that isn't nice and not to do that again, or I will tell."

At this point, you still might want to hover over your child and go to school the next day to inform the teacher what happened, but you know it's more important not to at this time. Instead, you focus on praising your child because you are proud of how they handled themselves. This tells your child that you care about what happens to them, but they can also take care of themselves. It also gives them the confidence to know how to handle people who are mean to them compassionately and politely.

Another way we can find ourselves hovering over our children is by not giving them enough space. This not only includes independent playtime, but the freedom to make mistakes, picture out what happened, and learn from them. Toddlers will need a little guidance when it comes to figuring out their mistakes and learning how to change their behavior or actions, so the error doesn't pop up again. Helping your child in this way is not hovering. You start to approach when you stop your child from making a mistake.

Make Problem-Solving a Positive Experience

Everyone runs into problems daily. We all have issues we need to solve. We might not always see them as problems, but they are there. Take time to reflect on your days and notice what problems occur in your life. Then, think of your toddler's days and their struggles. Picture out ways that you can turn everyone's problem-solving experience into more fun and favorable situation. For instance, if your child comes to you with a problem, look at them and say, "I see your problem.

Why don't we think of a couple of solutions together to help solve this problem?" With your toddlers, you can also make this into a game. For example, if they like Sherlock Holmes, they can play Sherlock, and you can be Watson trying to solve a problem.

Do-It-Yourself Projects

There are tons of do-it-yourself type projects for people of all ages. While your child can help you with home improvement projects at times, there are also smaller projects that you can work on with your child. You don't need to make sure that you do everything correctly or don't ask for help. Your child is going to learn more about solving their problems by watching you solve yours. Therefore, if they see you ask for help, they will understand that everyone asks for help. If your child sees you make a mistake, they will know that they can make a mistake, and everything will be okay.

Along with these types of projects, you can also look into puzzles. By the age of four, your child has probably put together tons of puzzles, which is a way that helps them problem solve. Continue to buy your child puzzles, but make sure that they are age-appropriate.

Problem Solving By Ages

One-Year-Old Problem-Solving Skills

While one-year-olds who are closer to two might start helping you put puzzles together or shapes in the correct spot, most of their skills are going to happen through observation. Have you ever stopped to think about how often a one-year-old will sit and watch other people? This is because the primary way they learn and start to develop their skills is through observing, listening, and taking in what is going on around them. At the same time, their mind is busy processing all the information they are taking in.

One of the best ways to help your one-year-old develop problem-solving skills is by showing them how to do something. For example, your child received new stackable blocks from your sibling. At first, they look at the blocks and seem puzzled. They might pick up a block and observe it more closely. At that moment, they don't understand that the blocks are meant to be stacked on top of each other. Therefore, you will take the time to show your child how the blocks work. Once you do this, hand the blocks over to your child and watch them mimic your actions. It's always an adventure to see how your young child catches on to what you have shown them so quickly!

Problem-Solving Activities

- Play a variety of accessible games for one-year-old children that will build their problem-solving skills, such as blocks and puzzles

- Playing peek-a-boo.

- Use objects to play hide-and-seek. You want your child to find the item. They are learning that just because they can't see an object doesn't mean it doesn't exist.

Two-Year-Old Problem-Solving Skills

At two-years-old, the memory comes onto the stage and gives your child a whole new way to learn how to problem-solve. This is a great age to start to bring easy puzzles and games, which will help build your child's problem-solving skills. Just like a one-year-old, the most significant way two-year-olds are going to learn is through observing. The only difference is; they are going to remember what they saw for a longer time.

Your child wants to color. They have asked you to help them get their crayons, but you are in the middle of preparing supper, which means that your hands are greasy and full of food you don't wish to get on the drawer where the crayons stay. You tell your toddler, "Go ahead and open the drawer, and you can do it." At first, they look at you, at the drawer, and look at you again. They have never opened the drawer before, so they are a bit anxious about getting it open. You assure them that they will be able to open the drawer just fine. "Open the drawer as I do," you tell your child. They then walk to the drawer as you start to wash your hands. You know that they have only been able to shake and bang the drawer to open it. They have never opened it before, so you are preparing to help your child. However, your child surprises you, and perhaps themselves, as they pull the handle and open the drawer without too much of struggle. "Look at what you did, baby!" You exclaim as you clap with your child's excitement.

At two-years-old, your child will use their memory to think about ways to solve a problem. They will start to come up with solutions in their mind and then see if this solution works. This is often why two-year-old children will stare at the problem before they try anything. It's not because they are becoming frustrated or thinking about giving up. They are trying to picture out how the toy works. The best step you can take is to observe your child. Notice their facial expressions as they are thinking and get an understanding of their thought process. You will also want to keep them so you can ask them if they would like to help if they become frustrated.

Problem-Solving Activities:

- Teach your child how to play "Simon Says."
- Use words like "over," "under," and "above," as this will help your child picture out what these words mean. They are great words to use when your child is looking for a toy that might be under the table.

- Gets toys and puzzles that let your child sort pieces through shapes and colors.

Three-Year-Old Problem-Solving Skills

Three-year-old children will often show a look of focus, yet they will become frustrated. They will use memory to solve problems but are more prone to trial and error than a two-year-old child. This is because three-year-old children will try things their way more than through observation or with help from their parents. This is also one reason why many people say that threes are worse than twos. It's because your three-year-old toddler will try a variety of new and exciting problem-solving skills while you are in another room. You won't have a clue what they are getting themselves into until you walk into the place for the surprise.

CONCLUSION

Thank you for reading all this book!

Adults ought to build conditions that fulfill fundamental development needs for identity, competence, freedom, and compassion to raise responsible and productive children. They identify these "four paths" as the Circle of Courage. There is clear proof that the needs of the Circle of Bravery are based on fundamental ideas, and perhaps even on the human DNA:

1. Relating: The child's need for human attachment is nurtured in confidence partnerships so that the kid can believe in "I am cherished."

2. Mastery: Training to deal with the environment boosts the child's inborn appetite for information, and the kid can say, "I will excel."

3. Independence: Increased responsibility nurtures the child's free will so the child can believe "I am in charge of my life."

4. Kindness: The essence of the infant is nurtured by empathy for all, such that the infant will say, "I have a life meaning."

In Western society decades, parents sought to raise decent children by teaching them to be compliant. Adults that claim compliance will set minimum standards, determined by the level of loyalty. Both children require people surrounding them who are compassionate, supportive, committed, and trustworthy if they are to thrive entirely. We have to become the immediate family of ancestors and parents that once encircled every boy.

You have already taken a step towards your improvement.
Best wishes!

Montessori at Home

Turn Your Home into Montessori

Written By

Jennifer Siegel

Table of Contents

INTRODUCTION

Thank you for purchasing this book!

Speak Positively, But Praise the Effort More Than the Child

They also hear less praise. And since these children tend to listen to fewer words in general, these negative expressions end up having a greater weight in their cognitive development. What will it be like repeatedly to hear that you never do anything, right? It's a problematic child environment to overcome. The difference between prohibition words ('do not do it,' 'stop') and encouragement ('very well') is excellent. It causes stress in the brain to hear them repeatedly. It is necessary to try to change orders for a more productive conversation.

Accountability comes with independence, and it needs to be remembered that the child is still learning its ability to control itself and think. Parents need to be very careful. And if we are honest, it's a significant challenge, and sometimes you need

9

simplify your life to take full advantage of parentage and be ready for parents emotionally.

makes sense to take Montessori into our home as a lifestyle. There are minor improvements that we can prepare without problems or difficulties in our habits and the way we support the child's growth. Harmony and joy are contained in the essence of life and the moments of our day. It is also wise for us to know more about being the mother/father of Montessori, the developmental stages of the child, and how he viewed the world, and how the atmosphere around us should be ready and prepared.

Enjoy your reading!

Cooperation

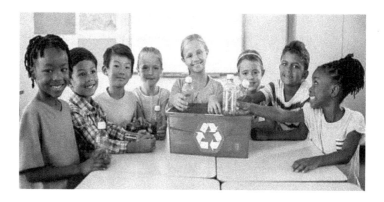

Cooperation can yield many prospects for the growth of the child, but it requires a lot of hard work and skill. You are cooperating with the child, who is just a toddler and needs your affectionate companionship at all costs. You cannot be robust, neither you can induce horrific compulsions among them. But in all ways possible, you have to nourish the fundamentals of care and start by listening to them. You can observe their notions, and you can stay connected with their memories in the long run. However, the question arises that what can be the possible ways to induce cooperation in the children? Well, the answer is as follows:

Ways To Be Cooperative With The Kids

ollowing Are The Ways To Be Cooperative With Your Kids

Taking turns

'hile we are taking turns, we are boosting team management and cooperation nong the toddlers. We need to understand that the baby is all growing up, and e is imitating the notions of all the elders in a respected manner. He needs to nderstand that while growing up, the life pattern can be hazardous, and the one, ho can become cooperative and compassionate, can only yearn to be successful. n example can be portrayed here to understand the thinking of the child. While e is playing blocks and or creating a puzzle, let him do his modes alternatively. ou have to take turns while you are building blocks for them, and then you have) see what he does in return. So, taking turns means that you have to be a team layer, and you have to do all the possible ways to become lenient to them.

'herefore, taking turns means that you have to be a team player and have to be ooperative with them at all costs.

. Explain your reasons for limits and reasons

A controlled environment is very pertinent to reflect good progress in society. It s the only way through which success and sustainability can be achieved in the eam. He is the sole benefactor of this process, and you have to make sure that e follows all the rules of the house. In this way, the house will be in order, and

12

he will be able to perceive management and demand perpetually. Therefore, th model of cooperation can be beneficial for the soul and heart of the child, an you need to induce this method in all ways necessary.

3. Take time to problem solve

You have to take time to see if the kids can solve the dilemmas that come in his lif Problems like the breaking of a glass, the absence of any material, and the overall los of any prodigal thing can be termed as examples. Thus, when such dilemmas appea the parent has to ask many minutes and the right questions to the child. Like wha seems to be the problem, baby, how can the problem be solved, is there any possibl solution to it? If so, then what can the alternative to it. When the child can find th answers, and if the answers are polite and keen, then please do encourage. Thi encouragement will give collective clout to the children, and hence, the child will b able to yield more love for the parent.

4. Do chores together start at an early age!

You have to encourage your child to do chores with you mentally. This means that if you are washing the dishes, then you must allow your child to share the burden of work with you. Bring your child into the work as well. Moreover, any obligation of a work, which i being conducted and shared by you, must be allowed to be executed by your child as well In this way, the child will learn how to cooperate with the parent and will come one step oser to the field of house-living. If you do not do it and do not allow the child to host ou; correctly, then you will see negative results of his upbringing. Therefore, you must e your child get the very best of housework and do all your best in making the child ok more clean and efficient.

. Giving more praise for cooperative efforts

f your child is doing something cooperative, then do please him and give him thumbs p. Otherwise, he won't reconcile with you. The child can do a lot of work once he given a boost and some mental encouragement. He can thaw his weaknesses and an convert them into happiness. He can see the role of his efforts progressively and an make the uttermost of the house routine. If you see the cooperation of others, hen please do let your child learn the art of collaboration as well. Also, giving him nore praise will clear all the mental barriers in his head about parenting, and he will ome one step near you in all possible ways. Therefore, more recognition can lead our child to the cooperation he deserves.

. Always be suggestive

Never be compulsive or orderly to your children. Always look to it that they have caring parent that is suggesting them to do more and more things. If you find a nistake in them, then do correct them genuinely and never let any other things come in the way. Once you will do bad things for the child, then ultimately, you will come in the ends and clouts of the issues. Your child will become paranoic and you will make a mess of your lifestyle. Therefore, suggestions to your chil will always lead to more innocence and cooperation in the child.

7. Give your child choices while maintaining the rules

You are maintaining the order in your child, but at the same time, you wan them to be cooperative. So, under such circumstances, it is very pertinent tha you are suggestive to all the followers of your child and let the child be on the same path with you. For instance, before bed, if you want your child to be following the rules, then ask him politely that what have you brushed your teeth and are your diapers clean and tidy. These cute and innocent questions will liberate the child from tensions, and he will be in more cooperation with you at all costs.

8. Talk your child about his feelings and let him know yours

Talk your child about the surface; he can witness and let him know the prospects of it as well. Let him see how he can communicate it with you and how you will transform yourself within limits. The child can harness more potential in this sense and will tell you about his progress in any field. He will come to know about the possibilities of life and will be very close to you in any regard. Therefore, ways be communicative with your child and never allow any emotional sturbance to impede your affiliation.

Explain them the situations in a calm manner

xplain to them the reasons why low expectations come in the way. And do not ell at them while you are doing so. If by chance, they are not able to clear any xam, then it is not your obligation to defame then or be obscurantist in front of hem. Just be a kind parent and let them understand the possibilities of life in an ffectionate manner. Try to suggest more cooperative tactics that will enable them ɔ yearn enjoyment. Therefore, the explanation of challenging situations in an asy way will make your child more cooperative and substantial.

0. Play games with them

Games like cricket and football are excellent games to boost creativity and subjectivity n the kids. If you hold a bat and hit your child ball with a good intellect and intent, then he child will learn cooperation by all means necessary. Even if you are playing the game ɔf football with him and you are running alongside him and telling him how to kick, hen you are cooperative, and the child will be more productive to your advice and earning. Therefore, play as much of the games, you want to play with him, and in the nd, you will end up being very affectionate with him. This is one of the most influential und splendid methods in making the child know the cooperation platform, and you should feel proud if you are doing so.

11. Always ask permissions before joining

Always ask permission to your child if you are about to join them and see what the child can do. If your child is playing the match of cricket and you are watching him, then try your best in not disturbing them; if you are washing the dishes and the child is watching movies, then ask his permission to join him. These examples assert your cooperative and affectionate behavior with the child and, eventually lead the child to a better end. However, if you are arrogant and stubborn enough to scold him vociferously, then you must not expect any kind of cooperation from the child. Because the child will be very stubborn for you, and he will not learn the art of collaboration.

12. Sharing is caring

If you are a busy guy and have a strict schedule on your time, then try your best to comply with your child. Understandably, the child will not get your routine and with innocent questions and a jolly mood, everybody can calm down. For instance, the child can get to the bottom of your practice. You are having a tough time dealing with him, so in such a circumstance, you must adhere to all the disciplinary steps that can navigate obedience in your child, and hence, you need to share things with him to achieve cooperation from his side. Therefore, he can care for you if you can share your routine with him.

So, with such ways and measures, the term cooperation can be easily put forward to the students and children as well.

Hacks To Get Through Those "Terrible Twos."

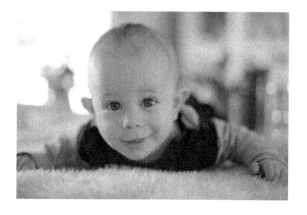

No matter how many "how-to" books you read or how long you spend surfing the web for ways to reign in your little demon child, there are inevitably going to be days where it will be challenging to deal with your toddler's moods and actions. Perhaps instead of scolding them for their behavior, you should take the time to take a closer look at the way you are parenting. Probably, it is time for a bit of change. These tips will help you triumph over those "terrible twos."

Having parenting hacks under your belt can make a massive difference between wanting to strangle or snuggle your child. The years of raising a toddler are when most of these tips are desperately needed the most. So here you have it!

Organization Techniques

aving kids means picking up, organizing, putting away, and cleaning A LOT of
ndom stuff. Here are some much-needed organization hacks to keep your
utter at bay.

Purchase an over-the-door shoe organizer and place over your child's door. This
can help store various toys in the clear pockets, which provide you easy-to-see
and grab access without stepping on gadgets that would otherwise be all over the
floor.

It may take a while, but sort out toy blocks, sort play things by color, and
others. This can be done in plastic bins.

Utilize wall storage to its full advantage to avoid having so much clutter upon
your floors to step on.

Store toys and art supplies in transparent containers, so they are easy to find.

Spend a bit of money on space-saving stacking storage bins.

Find activity tables or other kids furniture that also has built-in storage

Maximize space within the corners of your home with corner furniture and
bookcases that you can put bins in.

Welcome yourself to the world of chalkboard paint. Having a wall where your
kids can draw will hopefully keep them from adding crayon art pieces on
other walls within your home.

- If you happen to come across milk crates, grab them. They are ample storage as well as a brilliant pop of color.

- Utilize that old planter hanger to put stuffed toys inside.

- Use a pegboard for toy storage.

Maintaining Toys

Even though your toddler doesn't care too much about their favorite doll's hair being frizzy and knotted, take the time after playtime to clean-up their toys. Toys nowadays are quite expensive, so taking care of them will ensure that they will last longer and provide many more playtime hours.

When Going Shopping

Many parents dread taking their children to public places such as the grocery or clothing store. They always insist on buying something for them. A cute hack to minimize the demand is to tell them to take a photo of the item they desire so that it can be sent to Santa. This way, you will have lots of good gift ideas!

Potty Training

It is a real headache for some parents, the process of potty training. Some toddlers are merely afraid of the toilet, while others want to explore the bathroom. To process a bit easier, here are tips:

- Aiming for Cheerios – Put Cheerios in the toilet bowl and have your son aim for them. This is fun for him, but they will learn how to pee in the toilet at the same time.

- Cover public toilet sensors – Many kids freak the heck out when the automatic toilets flush in public restrooms. To aid this, stick a Post-It note over the sensor.

- Hang up toilet rolls backward – If you have a toddler that continually attempts to unwind the entire roll of toilet paper, install it back. This makes it much harder for them to accomplish that goal.

- Put up a "do not pass" sign under roll – Utilizing visual aids always is an excellent way of teaching your kids certain things. This goes for how much toilet paper they need to use too.

- Create a progress chart – When your child successfully goes to the bathroom without creating a mess, let them receive a sticker for their success.

- Buy and use puppy potty training pads – These suckers come in handy! Just put them under the sheets of your child's bed, so that way, if they have an accident, you can peel off the pad and throw the sheet in the laundry. If they do have an accident, have them help you in cleaning it up. This will help them realize that this is what has to happen when they have an accident.

- Bribery – No shame in bribing your toddler a bit to use the potty. Bribe them with big rewards at first, such as ice cream or a toy, and gradually decrease the bribes once they start getting the hang of going potty on their own, suc

as jelly beans or M&M's.

- Panty liners – These can come in handy if your child has occasion:

  accidents or have been properly potty trained but leak now and then.

Chore-Time

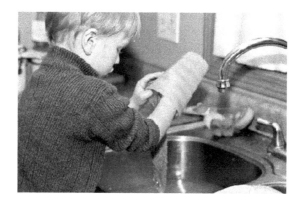

While your toddler-aged child cannot help with everything that needs cleaning

encourage them to help you. Please give them a damp cloth to wipe down thing

that are at their level. This helps them feel involved with the things you do and

helps them learn the power of responsibility as they get older and can help with

bigger chores.

While On The Go

here are quite a few toddlers who continuously demand to be held and carried, pecially when walking. They are more than capable of walking themselves. So ake a game out of it. Tell them to pretend that they are pushing you up the reet. They will have fun and forget that they are walking by themselves.

Mealtime

- Toddlers are pretty messy little eaters, so the average bib will probably not cover them completely. Instead of throwing old T-shirts away, save them to use during dinner time. Slip a shirt over their head to protect their clothes. Take off when they are done eating and wash with other clothing. This is an excellent tip if you are eating out in public and cannot go home and change clothing.

- Involving your child in meal prep will get them more excited to eat what you are preparing instead of stirring it around and playing with it.

- If your child tries new foods or eats items such as broccoli without spitting it out, reward them!

- Offer certain foods in different forms. Some people do not like cooked carrots but enjoy them raw.

- Make your child a little "food detective." Assist them in exploring their food by smelling it, licking it, or playing with it a bit.

- Occasionally, make dinner time an outdoor festivity. Changes in scene will make mealtime more exciting.

- Allow your kids to whip up a dinner menu. Inform them what they w— be having and let them engulf themselves in creating a colorful list. Th— will make mealtime seem like more of a fun event than a drab part of tl— routine.

- When planning meals, make sure to ask your children what they wou— like to consume. They will feel connected and a part of your me— planning.

- Play some music during dinner time. If you are eating Italian food suc— as pizza, let some Italian tunes play in the background. This helps i— making the content and not wanting to leave the table, as well as provide— valuable insight into another culture.

<u>TV Time</u>

While toddler-appropriate television shows can indeed help your child learn quit— a bit about their world, watching TV should be limited. A neat little trick I hav— learned is to have them start viewing a show in the middle of its showing— Toddlers cannot follow plotlines well anyways. So, it may seem like they got thei— television binge time in, but it was shortened. Parenting win!

Bedtime

he sleep patterns of your toddler can be somewhat of a nightmare in itself. Even
e tiniest bumps in the regular schedule can throw them off when it comes to
ing to bed and sleeping.

- Pick out a goodnight song – Ask your child about picking out a theme
  that can be sung each night before hitting the hay. The music you choose
  should be relaxing, and you can personally sing it or have it play on your
  phone.

- Practice mindfulness – Mindfulness for adults, requires a bit more work,
  but mindfulness as a whole is quite simple. Teach your toddler to observe
  how they feel and picture themselves in a peaceful place, such as floating
  along with the clouds. This will ultimately teach them to truly appreciate
  the comfort of lying in their bed in a dark room.

- Choose a bedtime best friend – I know as a child I loved my soft blanket.
  It was an object of pure comfort and always helped me sleep. Work with
  your child to pick a toy or other comfortable object to sleep with. And
  reserve that item for bedtime.

- Encourage plenty of physical activity before bedtime – This will help
  your child become tired and ready for bed.

- Create a relaxing bedroom environment – Ensure that before your child
  goes to bed, make it a habit that they clean up their room before climbing

into bed. It is also essential to keep rooms fresh at night; 65–70 degree

is excellent. You can use fun lamps, blackout curtains, and fans to g

your kid's room colorful, dark, and cold for ultimate sleepy time succes

As a parent, your child must see that you are happy because they can take awa

the smallest of body language. When the times are frustrating, and the going get

tough, take note of the following:

- Have a good sense of humor. When your toddler is going through thos

  phases where you want to pull your hair out, laugh. Just laugh a little! It i

  the best medicine in these situations.

- Take the time to slow down and enjoy even the smallest of moments.

- Appreciate the small things like your toddler does – the leaves, the bugs

  the rocks, the trees, etc.

- Always trust your judgment and gut feeling. Do you! Be confident ir

  raising your child.

- Take the time to remember that they are young human beings. Neve

  expect more from your toddler than they can appropriately deliver.

We are all human. There will be days that we mess up too. Do not get down or

yourself! Your young child is quite forgiving.

Dressing Themselves, Food Preparation, And Toilet Training

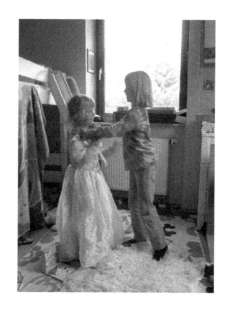

Routine is the gold standard in the toddler world, and most of the parenting that we

do occurs within the practice of routine daily maintenance. In these foundational

routines, you'll find the right structural balance to keep your toddler moving with the

rhythm of the household.

Getting Dressed

ith young toddlers, sometimes, the mimicry starts early! Evelyn has zero hair it loves to wave a hairbrush or my buzzing electric toothbrush over her head. ur daily dressing routines began to show in our toddlers' behaviors, with them tending arms and legs as shirts and pants are being put on.

ason was the easiest self-groomer, and we still joke about it today. This kid oke up every morning at 6 a.m. and came downstairs to our room wholly ressed. New underwear, jeans, shirt, socks, shoes, teeth brushed, hair combed— e whole enchilada. He was ready to go. Sure, he needed help to refresh his teeth r redo his hair occasionally, but he has his style and owns it.

s young as they are, kids may still have specific clothing needs thanks to sensory-lated issues or just plain old preferences (for our Ava, that meant nothing itchy d no denim, so welcome to Leggings-town!)

'his age group doesn't put up much of a fight. Without the agility and strength put on their clothes, they're at your mercy.

)ressing young toddlers in layers makes it easier to adjust to temperature changes s the day goes on.

)lder toddlers often become capable of getting themselves undressed for bath or ed, as well as getting dressed in simpler outfits. They'll also begin developing trong opinions on these outfits.

Choose accordingly. Once they're able to dress, consider outfits that match the abilities. Avoid buttons or tough zippers.

Be attentive. Being available (not preoccupied) and standing by your toddler while they dress is a great thing, but you should remind them that you're just there in case they need you.

Take time. When a toddler knows that you or your partner is in a hurry or need to get something done quickly, they'll resist and do the exact opposite. Try to give yourself plenty of time.

Regulating Your Own Emotions And Moods: Go Ahead, We'll Catch-Up

Toddlers don't know how to hurry, so rushing them will just frustrate you. Consider where you're running to. Can you be a few minutes late? When you choose calm, the whole family dynamic will follow suit.

Teachable Parent Tools To Deploy

Be a clothing buddy. Help your kids gain confidence and get dressed alongside them. I laid both of our outfits on the bed and put the pieces on, one by one with colorful commentary!

Prep your clothes. To plan, every Sunday, we do laundry. We also pull outfits for the week for everyone, with underwear, socks, and accessories included in small

etal bins labeled "Monday" through "Friday." The days are color coordinated
r the younger ones, so if we say "Mason, go get the orange bin," he knows it is
uesday.

When Hits The Fan

nce your toddler can dress and undress, it's best to give them no more than two
hoices. We allow the kids to help choose their outfits on Sundays for the week,
> there isn't a fight. If they're not feeling the clothes we chose, they can switch
ut the bin for a different day.

ho doesn't love eating? Well, when your little table-mate is tossing your
omemade pesto sauce to the dogs and offering you a slobbered-on hunk of garlic
read, you might think differently.

'm a veteran of food combat, and I've bounced back from serving spaghetti
narinara over a beige carpet. Despite the mess, eating is one of the most joyful
imes. Setting kids up to enjoy food and "eat the rainbow" now ensures they'll be
vell-rounded eaters later. Using the following tools to make eating fun, you'll
nake it less of a struggle for you and your littlest gourmet.

Eating

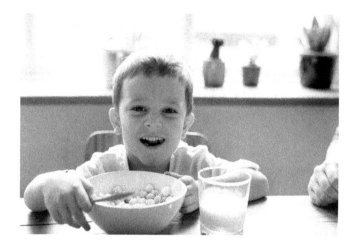

We all choose our parenting battles, and Jen and I decided it was important to u
to make sure our kids had developed palates. Even trying to raise little foodies
we still run into issues. Ava does not eat cheese, Charlie won't eat any leafy greens
and Mason won't touch avocados. Having a picky eater is a substantial universa
frustration, so what do you do? Remember, those small successes in thi
marathon help tremendously. It can be easiest to take the three or four foods you
toddler latches on to and continue to serve them, and there's a time and place fo
that route, but it's certainly not always. We decided to tackle this issue head-on.

Evelyn developed an oral aversion after being force-fed antibiotics, so she views
eating as intimidating. We're acclimating her by showing her it's a fun process, so
she's allowed to play with her food—feel it, squeeze it, and, yes, throw it. We talk
to her about "kissing" her fish crackers and raisins, so when she licks her lips, she

nderstands there's something right there. It is exhausting, for sure. But raising oddlers who have healthy palates will typically guarantee they won't be the adult :dering a steak and potato dinner "with no parsley and hold the salad."

our toddler doesn't understand that you're trying to help establish good eating abits—they only care about the frozen yogurt pop. They're more apt to partake they like what they see.

lost everything hits the floor at this stage. They do well with purées but keep nem progressing. Finger foods work best because toddlers get to feel them, and id-safe animal-shaped toothpicks are great for picking up food. But the first time our gleeful girl grabs a spoon or a kiddie fork, don't expect excellent results; :velyn uses her dirty fork to brush her hair.

hey're still getting the hang of chewing, so watch them closely. Food should be ite-sized for their mouth, not yours. Keep cubes (olives, chicken, broccoli) no irger than the size of your pinky nail. When babies are first experimenting, they at like little squirrels, "munching" with the front of their mouths, whereas oddlers learn to move food to the back and to chew.

Vith age comes skill and the use of a spoon or fork. Consider starting a healthy lialogue around food, aiming for specifics over generalities, like "This carrot will help you see in the dark," or, "This blueberry will give you a strong brain!" over "This is yummy!"

The amount of food you think they need may be very different from the amount of food they feel like they need. Start with tiny portions fit for little tummies and let them ask for more. It's best for kids to eat until they're full, not necessarily until they clear their plates.

Eat together if you can, sit down as a family every night. It doesn't matter if you have one kid or nine, or if you sit in the kitchen, at a picnic table outside, or around the coffee table. Just. Sit. Together. And serve your kids what you eat, at least for dinner.

Don't assume they won't like it. On a family cruise, we learned our kids were willing to try strange things and complex flavors: Ava loved chicken tikka masala, Charlie would eat any seafood, and Mason could devour spinach enchiladas. Don't cheat your tod out of exciting, necessary experiences by keeping menus limited.

Fly new food under the radar. If there are "tried and true" items on the plate, slipping in something new might go unnoticed. A nutritionist friend recently told us that anxiety causes an increase in stomach acid, leading to feelings of fullness. Having something familiar on the plate leads to less stress surrounding mealtime.

an't pinpoint a specific age for when it's appropriate to potty-train your kids—

s different for everyone. The best way to assess whether they are ready is by

ommunicating and reading their signals, which might include:

an they express when they're wet?

o they hold their diaper?

an they mimic your toilet use?

o they attempt to wipe while you're changing them?

re they drawn to a training potty or capable of sitting and staying on it?

<u>Toilet Training</u>

m not an expert; however, I'm a dad who's researched potty-training, worked in

e parenting space for a decade, and been through this rodeo four times.

cientifically speaking, a toddler between twelve and eighteen months has very

tle bladder control, so training them early isn't so much about teaching them,

's about training you.

ith our family, little hints were clutch. Evelyn cried every time she peed or pooped

her diaper, so her discomfort signaled to us that she's ready to transition. Mason

ttempted to use the potty on his own. They would also approach the adult potty and

ull at the seat or try and mimic our actions—standing up, sitting down, and drawing

n the toilet paper roll.

We've had two training potties; the first, a simple red seat "bowl" that sat low to the ground. Our second, a Fisher-Price sing-along version, played a song every time it was used, which encouraged them to keep using the potty.

The tricky part about being able to determine whether your kids are ready is to acknowledge their state of mind. The idea of sitting on a potty could be overwhelming (from a sensory perspective) or exciting (from an independence standpoint)—it's all uncharted waters.

She is acknowledging ownership over something as crazy as the potty can go long way. I like our Evelyn, and your Tod starts to approach the training potty you'll know she's almost ready to start training. Seeing Evelyn unroll yards of toilet paper is frustrating, but we know she's growing used to the bathroom's many moving pieces!

At this more advanced stage, disposable training pants like Pull-Ups help bridge the gap between being ready to potty-train but not having the control to hold it while sleeping.

Go for the stand-alone. A stand-alone potty with or without a dump-able (no pun intended) insert a must. We also purchased a smaller toilet seat insert that clips onto the regular one to keep smaller tushies from falling in.

op a squat, buttercup. We began by introducing our toddlers to the idea of sitting own on the potty to pee or poop. Pee was generally what happened first, but if e got a poop, bonus!

at first, potty second. Our pediatrician explains that when a toddler eats or inks, it can trigger their need to go to the bathroom. Consider using that timing get your little one used to use the potty.

Encouraging Good Toddler Behavior

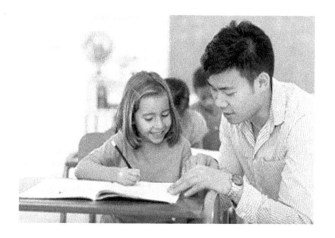

To encourage positive behavior in children is through praise. Children seek love and recognition for their efforts and progress. Praise increases children's self-confidence and motivation by making them feel happy. It's beneficial to give them confidence in their abilities and to show them that they feel proud when they behave correctly, thereby encouraging good behavior. Here are some highly useful tips to help promote positive action.

Encourage Effort

Use praise to encourage effort and to enhance the progress of your child. A child who can use the bathroom alone for the first time or perform a task deserves recognition. In this way it is encouraging the child's development and autonomy.

39

Reinforce Attitudes

njoy instilling some values that you consider fundamental, meaningful, and positive.
y praising and reinforcing attitudes, you help to develop social skills that will make
lationships easier in the future.

Praise The Effort, Regardless Of The Result

he effort must be praised even if the goal is not fully achieved. If your child did
ot receive an excellent grade, but studied and worked for this to be possible, it's
gnificant to recognize him. Praise is key to staying motivated and hence
nproving your bottom line.

Praise Good Behavior

's important to praise good behavior; don't save compliments only for
utstanding achievements. Small behavior improvements should also be valued.
f we only pay attention at times where action needs work, children will feel
nclined to do wrong.

Approve Or Disregard Attitudes And Not The Child

As much as you consider your child to be very handsome, intelligent, etc., avoid telling them this often. This type of label turns out to be as harmful as the opposite ("you're dumb," "you're bad," etc.). Try to mark your approval or disapproval regarding attitudes, not the child.

Value The Achievements Of The Family

It is significant to value the achievements and efforts of the family. If a child has accomplished something, it's important to praise them, as well, and accomplishments of the family members. It is beneficial to recognize the effort of all the elements and celebrate the achievements in the family.

Rewards

You can also choose to reward your child, such as a gift, a trip to the movies, or candy if you want to reinforce an attitude. But don't make it a routine because this can lead to only good behavior when rewarded. Most action should be awarded only by praise. Also, you may be tempted to use the allowance as a reward. We don't recommend it. Never use the funding to "buy" your child.

Rewarding the child for good behavior teaches them to understand that there is a direct link between action and consequence.

member that as a parent, you are a role model for your children. You must be good role model by providing them with appropriate rules and standards to low. Consistency is the key. Children learn by observing others, and they will rn these qualities. With a little persuasion and positive reinforcement, you can ich, encourage, and create positive behavior in children.

How To Stimulate Good Behavior In Children?

imulating good behavior in children is one of the best ways to impose limits, thout having to apply punishments continuously. The only problem is how to that. In most cases, our little ones tested our limits and seemed to do anything t to obey.

e the Example

eing an example is the most effective way we need to teach our children anything both good and bad. When it comes to encouraging good behavior in children, is no different. Here are a few examples of what you can do for your child to arn.

atch your child's attention when you split snacks with your husband or when ou have to wait in the bank queue, pointing out that adults also have to share nd stay too.

Realize The Good Behavior

If you are like any parent in the world, when your child is behaving well, you leave them playing alone and take advantage of the time to do anything you may need to. But when your child is misbehaving, you direct all your attention to them to resolve the situation. Your attention is what kids most want, so to get this attention. Sometimes children will misbehave. The best way to encourage good behavior in children is to pay attention when they are behaving well and to take your attention from them when they are misbehaving. This is completely counter-intuitive for us and can be a difficult habit to cultivate. But once you get used to it, it will become easier and more comfortable.

A great way to do this is to play with your child when they are quiet in their corner and praise them when they obey you the first time you speak.

Understand The Stage Of Development

This tip is easy to understand. Each child has a behavior; though, you cannot require a child of three to act as the same as a child that is ten. That is, do not try to go to a three-hour lunch with your little boy hoping they will be quiet for the whole lunch. Do not expect a two-year-old child to stop stuffing everything in their mouth. Each age has a phase, and it is no use wanting to demand different behavior from a child.

Have Appropriate Expectations

This is a continuation of the above tip. Parents have high expectations. This is not wrong when expectations are possible. For example, don't expect a tired child behave well, or a one-month-old baby to sleep through the night.

Create Structure And Routine

A child with a structured routine tends to behave better. They already know what to expect and are used to it. A child with a performance feels safe and thus lives more calmly. A child without a routine has a sense of insecurity that will disrupt much in the time to educate and encourage good behavior.

Uses Disciplinary Strategies

Rather than humiliating or beating children, there are positive disciplinary strategies that teach them the right things, set boundaries, and encourage good behavior in children. Some of these are: give options, put somewhere to think, talk, show affection, and a system of rewards (reward can be a simple compliment, it does not have to be gifts or food).

Understand That The Bad Behavior Worked So Far

If throwing tantrums and disobeying worked for them to get your attention so far, changing this behavior will take time. They will have to understand that you will no longer pay attention to them when they misbehave, but when they behave well.

Instilling acceptable behavior practices in young children is a must for an responsible parent, but sometimes it can also be quite complicated and laborious Although, beginning to instill this type of behavior as early as possible will help build a good foundation for the child's behavior and attitudes in the future. It necessary to be aware that in the first years of life, the children are like "sponges, and results will be better if you begin to show them early and direct them to appropriate behaviors of life in society.

More ideas to help parents with the task of encouraging good behavior in their children

Models To Follow

Children tend to mirror the behaviors of parents and those with whom they coexist more closely. So, be careful about your actions and language when the child is around to avoid misunderstanding ideas and misconceptions about how you should behave towards others. This includes talking properly and conducting politely to both your partner and family, as well as to the child. Try to avoid loud, unstructured argument when the child is around. We do not mean you can't disagree with your spouse because the child must also be aware that these exist. But try to have the arguments always controlled and civil around children.

e Firm

arents should be affectionate, but still adamant about instilling discipline in their ildren. The child must know how to respect their parents, even when they do not ave what they want. Understanding when to say "no" at the right times is a gnificant step in your education.

ositive Body Language

our body language has a huge impact when you are trying to instill a specific behavior children. Given the height of the child, a parent standing while correcting the errors d applying discipline is often viewed as authoritative. It is advisable to place yourself the same level as the child's eyes. Sit next to the child while talking to them and always aintain eye contact.

stablishing Limits

is fundamental to establish limits, rules, and consequences for unwanted ehavior. Increase limits on children to be able to distinguish right from wrong. hey need to know what is not acceptable and transparent reasons that make it rong so that there is no doubt in the child's mind about the behavior to adopt.

ou started tracking your child's progress long before they left the warmth of your belly: 1 the tenth week, the heart began beating; on the 24th week, their hearing developed nd listened to your voice; in the 30th week, they began to prepare for childbirth. Now hat they are in your arms, you're still eager to keep up with all the signs of your little one's development and worries that they might be left behind. Nonsense! Excessive worry won't help at all, so take your foot off the accelerator and enjoy each phase. Your child will realize all the fundamental achievements of maturity. They will learn to walk, talk, potty, and when you least expect it, they'll be riding a bicycle alone (and no training wheels!). They will do all this in time.

Stop taking developmental milestones so seriously. For example, your 7-month-old son will be able to sit alone, and at age three, will be able to ride a tricycle. Consider what is expected for each age just for reference. The best thing to do is to set aside the checklist of the abilities your child needs to develop and play together a lot. There is no better way to connect with and build your child than through playtime.

To help you even further in realizing the goals mentioned above or processes, would like to say some tips here that stimulate a child's intellectual, motor, social and emotional development:

How Parents and Caregivers can Unleash the Native Intelligence in Toddlers

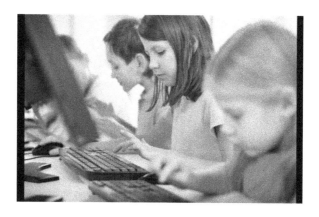

Modern US child-rearing, with its over-emphasis on containing and directing children, is moving further and further away from nurturing the essential aspect of intelligence in young children: initiative, attention, concentration, persistence and self-control. At this time, in the United States in 2015, there is also a very unconstructive pressure to emphasize academic work with young children despite research showing that doing so is harmful.

ou can raise your child more simply, with higher regard, less stress, and better utcomes. What you need to do differently is to give your child plenty of opportunities to practice these skills.

urturing your young child's intelligence is not about drilling them on their umbers or taking them to piano lessons. Instead, as often as possible, given free ein to their instincts to explore and learn. As long as they are engaged in an ctivity that is not destructive, trust that they are learning something they need to now, even if it's hard for you to imagine what it is. If they're working hard at omething, they are developing their initiative, the focus of attention, oncentration, self-control, and persistence.

Nurture initiative. As your child starts to walk, they can explore the world more ully, which understandably creates more work and worry for the parents. As your hild becomes a toddler, you will get lots of advice to give them choices and to mit the options. For example, if you feel it's essential for them to eat veggies ith their meal, you might ask whether they would like green beans or salad with heir lunch.

Nurturing initiative is about giving choices, but it's more than that. Let's take the xample of a child who wants to work in the sandbox. He may appreciate the texture. Ie may be learning about the conservation of volume.

Do not feel you must continuously guide, direct, or entertain your toddler. That will lead you to do so much for your toddler that their initiative never gets an opportunity to come out to play.

How does the child respond when we don't allow them to do things on their initiative? Sometimes they become very frustrated and throw a tantrum. Over time, many of them become passive and quit trying to initiate anything, merely waiting for direction from adults all the time. That will keep them from becoming the capable, self-reliant, fully-realized person they were born to become.

To nurture their intelligence, support their initiative whenever you can. Trust that they know what they need to learn, and they will work hard to understand it if only we don't interfere.

2. Nurture focused attention and concentration. Twenty years ago, I worked as consultant to 12 Head Start classrooms. I thought it was pretty impressive how the teachers kept the children's attention and kept them from getting into trouble. I could see that having all the children focus on the teacher all the time meant that some children were bored, and others weren't keeping up. But, that's how school was, and I thought it was the best we could do with toddlers and their short attention spans.

At that time, I had no awareness of how much we interrupt children's concentration. Believing that toddlers have short attention spans, I thought that

eping them too preoccupied with getting into trouble was the best we could do
r them.

Iow I know that toddlers can demonstrate relatively high levels of attention and
oncentration, focusing on something interesting for 20- 30- 40 minutes. But we
ave to let them. What does that look like?

oddler raking leaves. This kind of work is both challenging and beneficial for a
oddler, requiring the focus of attention, concentration, self-control, and
ersistence.

) Let them follow their interests. When we're interested in something, it holds
   our attention. Toddlers want to do what other people can do, so their
   interests naturally lead them to work on essential skills. Note whatever work
   interests them, putting their shoes on and off, pouring water or sand from
   one container to another, doing and redoing a puzzle 30 times. As long as it's
   not destructive, why not let them work at it? When they're working at
   something they're interested in, they're developing the part of their brain that
   manages attention, and that's essential brain development!

) Reduce clutter. Neither children nor adults concentrate well in cluttered
   environments. You can support your child's developing attention by keeping
   minimal amounts of toys in their environment. Think about reducing noise
   distractions, too. For example, break the habit of leaving the TV on.

c) Hold yourself back from interrupting their concentration. When your toddler is working at something that is challenging and requires concentration, notice that and refrain from talking. When we talk, toddlers stop everything from paying attention to the person and the language. We may be able to talk and drive and put on our lipstick all at the same time. But a toddler can't. If they're concentrating on something, like a puzzle, support their brain development by remaining quiet.

3. Nurture persistence. The past suggestions apply to the continuation, too. People of all ages persist more at learning when they are interested in the work and when they chose the profession. Nurturing initiative helps to promote persistence.

a) Be conscious about not interrupting them when they're working at something.

b) Give them time. Toddlers need a lot of time to work at things that are very quick for us to do. I have seen toddlers take 30 minutes to clean the table before lunch. All that time, they're developing their brains and their ability to persist at something. If we give them time, they will learn to endure.

Most schools get this wrong. They ring the bell every 50 minutes to change classes or activities. For many children, it's about the point they're just starting to understand something that adults intervene to change actions. Many of those children give up and quit trying in those classes. To give your toddler more

53

portunity to develop persistence, find ways to provide them with time to keep orking at something until they picture it out.

Get comfortable with errors and mistakes, and let your children learn from their own mistakes. Most of us grew up learning from an early age that mistakes are embarrassing and are to be avoided. But that's not a constructive attitude; we never know anything if we're not willing to make mistakes.

We need to be careful not to communicate our anxieties and discomfort about eir errors. If they're struggling with something challenging, we can simply sit on ir hands and demonstrate confidence that they can work it out. If it's too hard day, maybe they can do it better tomorrow. They will be better able to persist we let them learn from their own mistakes and hold ourselves back from tervening.

Nurture self-control. All of the recommendations above support the evelopment of self-control. Let your toddler initiate and work at whatever terests them, whenever you can, and they will work in a self-motivated way and rect themselves. Let them learn from their own mistakes, and they will correct emselves. They will know so much more in the process.

ike every other skill a person develops, toddlers need to practice with self-ontrol. Look for opportunities to let your child practice with managing their npulses and body. Sit on your hands when they are engaged in constructive ork.

The real preoccupation of toddlers is to develop the skills of more mature people. When possible, we need to give them opportunities to control themselves because that supports their development of essential skills.

Some Tips To Unleashing Your Child's Creative Potential

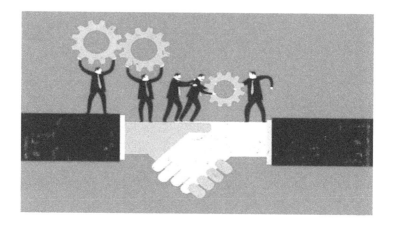

Creativity is the demonstration of transforming new and smart thoughts into truth. Imagination is characterized by the capacity to comprehend the part in modern manners, reveal mystery patterns, connect disconnected marvels, and produce reactions. Creativity involves methods: thinking, at that point, creating. Inventiveness is a combinatorial power: it's our ability to take advantage of our 'internal' pool of sources – data, understanding, data, proposition, and the entirety of the pieces populating our psyches. Innovativeness implies being fit for concocting something new.

ke this, imaginative reasoning is the ability to remember anything. Imagination a scaffold to examining. While your baby is creative and curious, she will think answers to the difficulties she experiences, similar to how to hold the square nnacle from falling. Imagination permits your baby to come to be a great, allenging, and sure student later on, while she begins school. One of the most werful fundamental strategies that your newborn child is checking out her novativeness is by a method of trying different things with the work of art aterials. As she gets that thick colored pencil and gets to works of art, you will e her craftsmanship and composing exchange and rise as extra controlled and lvanced as she develops. For amazingly more youthful children, work of art and ew composing abilities are one and the equivalent. It's everything about scovering what pastels can do with these cool things. At that point, your infant nds the connection among her hand holding the pencil and the street she made n the website page: Presto! Consider how intriguing this must be for her! She ould now be able to make a real "mark" on the world. This hop in deduction apacities is helped close by her new ability to protect things in her fingers and ms. The creating control your youngster has over the muscle tissues in her ngers lets her pass a marker or paintbrush in light of a thought process and an bjective.

What Is The Creative Mind??

Inventiveness implies glancing in another manner at something. It is th importance of "examining outside the edge." Imagination on this sensatic frequently includes what is considered horizontal addressing or the capacity t see drifts that are not evident.

Examination

Sooner than pondering innovatively about something you initially have for yo to get it. This requires the ability to investigate matters cautiously to realize wha they infer. Regardless of whether you're taking a gander at a book, a recordset, a exercise plan, or a condition, it would be best to examine it first.

Liberality

Imagination includes addressing things differently inside the setting of th question. It would help if you separated any presumptions or predispositions yo can have and watch matters in another way. Utilizing going to an issue with ope considerations, you permit yourself the danger to think innovatively.

Association

This may appear to be nonsensical: aren't creative individuals recognized fo being muddled? Endeavor is an essential piece of inventiveness. At the same time as you would potentially need to get a bit chaotic while endeavoring out anothe ought, you at that point need to set up your arrangements so others can have

e option to secure and follow-through along with your creative and wise. Being

for structure, a game-plan with clean dreams, and time limits are essential.

orrespondence

ople will handiest regard your inventive idea or arrangement if you may talk it effectually

the individuals you work with or on your clients or organizations. In this way, you have

have substantial composed and oral discussion capacities. Moreover, you may need an

cellent method to comprehend a situation before intuition innovatively around it. In

is way, you additionally may be a broad audience. Utilizing posing the correct inquiries

d ability in a difficult situation could offer you an exciting response.

<u>Various Stages Of Child's Creativity</u>

here are four scopes of drawing and composing for tiny children that you can

e as your infant develops from 15 months to three years of age. The word that

e plans recorded underneath is rough; your child may likewise ace those abilities

eedier or increasingly slow to develop simply high-caliber. Development

oesn't show at an equivalent speed for each youngster. Through providing

hashed fun encounters with an implication of craftsmanship and composting

aterials, you will see forward improvement throughout the years.

Stage 1: Scripting Spontaneously 15 Months To 2½ Years

This is when small kids regularly realize that their motions add to the lines ar scrawls they see on the page. Such scribblings are generally the aftereffect expansive hand motions with the colored pencil or pencil in the kid's clench han There's bliss in creating work of art at all ages. However, at this level, especiall numerous children relish the comments they're getting from their faculties: Th sound of the pastel, the aroma of the chalk, the softness of the earth. For variou youngsters, this tactile information can be excessively, and they may now nc appreciate some craftsmanship sports at this degree like finger-depict. As the create to endure vast physical knowledge, you could steadily re-bring work of a exercises into their collective.

Stage 2: Structured Scribbling 2 Years To 3 Years

As youngsters create higher oversees over the bulk of their palms and palms, the scrawls begin to exchange and end up extra controlled. Children may mak rehashed blemishes on the page—open circles, skewed, bent, or even vertica strains.

Stage 3: Patterns and Lines 2½ Years To 3½ Years

Children currently consider that composing is made of strains, bends, an rehashed styles. They attempt to mirror this of their book. So Simultaneously, a they won't write real letters, you can see added substances of letters in thei

awing. These could be bends, circles, and bends. That is an exciting time as
ur little child understands that his delineation passes on importance! As an
casion, he may likewise record something after which mentions to you what
ate it says. This is an essential advance towards dissecting and composing.

age 4: Images Of Objects Or People 3 Years To 5 Years

umerous grown-ups consider "pix" a picture of something. This ability to keep a
oto on your contemplations, after which comprises it on the site page, is a
asoning aptitude that sets aside some effort to create. In the first place, Kids call
eir developments impromptu. This implies they end the image and afterward name
eir work of art with the names of people, creatures, or devices they're acquainted
ith—those alterations after some time. Before long, you'll see your newborn child
ranging before drawing what he will make. Likewise, you will observe additional
omponents inside the pictures, higher control in how your youngster handles the
astel or marker, and utilizations other hues. What else to be looking for? Youngsters'
rst depictions as often as a possible form of circles. You could see a sun—an unusual
ng, with a lot of stick "beams" taking pictures out—or somebody usually a hover
ith generally conspicuous human highlights. When your little child has begun to
raw pix deliberately, she has aced representative reasoning. This important
chievement in pondering abilities moves toward that your kid realizes that strains on
aper can be an image of something different, similar to a habitation, a feline, or an
dividual. At this degree, your kid likewise begins developed to catch the qualification

among photos and to compose. You can also observe him. They draw an image and afterward jot a couple "words" underneath to depict what he has attracted or tell story. When your youngster is equipped to extend his story with you, he might be incited to "creator" progressively more works of art as he develops.

Stage 5: Letter And Word Practice 3 To 5 Years

Kids have needed to appreciate letters and print for quite a while at this point and are beginning to apply letters in their unique composition. Commonly youngsters start by utilizing exploring different avenues regarding the letters of their names as these are generally familiar with them. Furthermore, they make "imaginary letters" using duplicating regular letter shapes. They will usually envision that their completed letter must be genuine. It would appear that different letters they have seen all through this time, kids also start to recall how a couple of words are manufactured from images that can be shorter. A couple of words are produced using models that can be longer—accordingly, their scrawls exchange. As opposed to one long series of letters or letter-like shapes, your newborn child's composing currently has fast and long styles that appear words or sentences. Indeed, even as those letters and words are likely not, at this point, in fact, exact it does now not tally number. This energizing achievement implies that your infant is starting to comprehend that text and print have meaning.

Approaches To Strengthen Children's Creativity

xtricate up the controls. Infant care transporters who persistently control kids' mes practically decline immediacy and self-assurance, which can be essential to e inventive soul.

mpower diligence. The entirety of the innovative vitality inside the globe is futile the item isn't seen through to last little detail. Show gratefulness for kids' ideavors. Stifle the drive to perform commitments for youngsters.

ndure the "strange." Allow kids to understand that it isn't generally critical to ave the "precise" response to the issue – that novel, progressive, and new rocedures are esteemed.

)ffer an innovative environment. Creative materials ought to be accessible to the outhful baby for his utilization. A few straightforward contraptions incorporate ooks, records, drawing substances, articles to make sounds with, dirt, and squares. Jnstructured toys and materials convey preschoolers with opportunities for nvisioning and license the child to utilize gadgets in a determination of strategies. Be autious about demoralizing wandering off in fantasy land. Wandering off in fantasy ind is, beyond question, a symbolic way.

Speaking The Potty Language

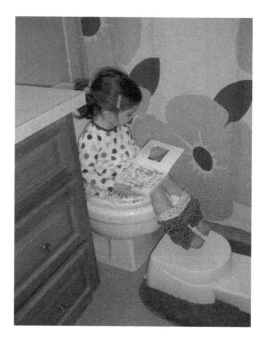

We talked on how to train your kids to use the potty let dive into speaking th

potty language.

I know what you're thinking, are there potty languages? How do you speak th

potty language? The fact is there are potty languages, and I'm going to show you

how to express those potty language. Still, first, you need to understand the fac

that the more natural you speak the word, the more relaxed your child feels with u teaching him how to use the potty, but to be honest, it not about the kinds words but it how we say them to our kids.

ow, most parents make mistakes of using the potty language to hurt their kids; ey say it in a much-intensified tone, which might result in kids being ashamed d embarrassed about themselves.

ou need to learn the best style to communicate the potty language to your kids. he potty language is an essential aspect of potty training; if you're going to teach ur kids to use the potty, you also need to understand how to speak the potty nguage. Most families have their unique way of communicating the potty nguage with their kids. Still, I'm going to show you the best and suitable way to form the potty language with your kids better.

How To Speak The Potty Language To Your Kids?

ne of the best and suitable ways to speak the potty language to your kids is to:

Be Polite

you need to talk the potty language to your kids, you need to be polite, don't use e potty language against them, don't let your kids feel bad when you use the word ainst them. Be courteous when saying the potty language to them. You see, kids ve it when you speak to them politely. Most parents don't get on well when it comes potty training with their kids, and It is because they often make the mistake of using the potty language to hurt their kids. Don't worry, your kids, when saying th potty word because you make things difficult for yourself and your kids. When yo use the potty word against your kids, your kids might lose their interest in pot training, and it might frustrate you in the end because you wouldn't want all yo effort on potty training your kids to be wasted. Just be polite when saying the pot language to your kids.

Don't Get Too Harsh When Speaking the Potty Language

Now, it is similar to what I said earlier, but the truth is, speaking politely and no being harsh are different. When you talk politely, it involves your mouth, but no being harsh includes your actions towards kids. You need to understand that kid often watch how you react at them during potty training, and when you ar speaking the potty language, if you are too harsh on them when speaking th potty language, it might not end up well for both you and your kids. So, don't ge too loud.

Use Cute Slangs

Instead of using words like, "Tracy goes to the toilet," when she wants to poop, yo could use words like "Tracy, go poop on your potty." You get what I'm trying to do instead of saying it the matured way, use slangs to say it, but don't get me wrong I neve used a hurtful or abusive slang; I used a cute and straightforward slangs. Just make i simple when speaking the potty language, and also add a few slangs to it just for fun

Ensure Your Body Is Speaking The Potty Language

Now don't get me all wrong. I'm not telling you to say to your body, body, you need to start saying the potty language, well that isn't possible, but anyways what I meant is you demonstrating with your body when speaking the potty language. If you're going to talk about the potty language, you need to show with your hands and legs. Okay, let say, you have a kid, and she hurries to meet you and then tells you, "Mom, I want to poop," now if you're to reply her, you could demonstrate with your hands as you talk, you could point at the potty as you tell your kid to go poop on the potty. Demonstrations make potty training fast and, at the same time, help you speak the potty language to your kids. Kids better understand you when you demonstrate so that a few demonstrations wouldn't hurt you.

Ensure Your Kids Feel Comfortable When You Speaking The Potty Language

Now, not all kids love hearing the potty language; my sister's child is a victim of ; she doesn't like it when her mom says, "Tracy, go poop on your potty." Try making sure your kids are comfortable with you speaking the potty language, but don't get things twisted. The potty word is the best way to communicate with your kids during potty training. Still, for some kids they don't feel comfortable with it. Ensure your kids feel comfortable when you use the potty language to communicate with them during potty training.

Speak The Potty Language At The Right Time

It was one of my mistakes when I went into potty training with my little child and I believe it has happened to lots of parents. Most parent often makes the mistake of speaking the potty language always to their kids; the most parent often uses it to hurt their kids. In contrast, some parent loves making fun of the word. Still, you only speak the potty language during potty training, or if your kids give you the signal of wanting to go to the toilet. Again, you actually can't speak the potty language when your kids might be reading, or having fun, or doing something not related to potty training. You really can't say it. You're just going to hurt them the more. Just watch the time you speak the potty language, so you won't end up hurting your kids.

All right, guys. I do hope It was helpful to you, and I do hope you understood everything I explained, and believe me, if you do implement them, they're going to work well for you.

So, as I said earlier, speak the potty language at the right time, now it might not look much to you, it means a lot, which is why I'm going to show you the best time to speak the potty language with your kids what I'm about to show you help guide you on when to talk about the potty language to your kids.

The Best Time To Speak The Potty Language To Your Kids

The best time to speak the potty language is;

er 1: During potty training

er 2: When your kids give you a sign or signal of wanting to go to the toilet

er 3: When your kids make use of the potty

er 4: When your kids communicate with you using the potty language

er 5: When your kids see you making use of the toilet

Now all these are the best and appropriate times to speak the potty language with our kids. Just make sure when you are telling the potty language to your kids, they are comfortable and show interest in it.

So, we've talked on the best time to use the potty language, so what is the potty language? I know that you're asking yourself right now, but not to worry, I'm going to show you.

Potty Language

What I'm about to list might sound a little bit silly and crazy and wacky but b

meaningful to you and your kids

All right, so these are just a few examples of the potty language, but let me tell you a

little secret when you use a particular language during potty training with your kids

and they feel comfortable with that language, that is the potty language your kid.

better understand. So, try figuring out also which language your kids do understanc

during potty training.

Kids Sign Language For Potty Training

Potty Sign

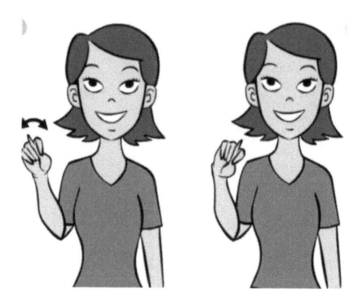

Turn your hand into a fist and ensure your thumb is peeking out between the index and central finger.

Also, ensure your fist is out and try shaking it around for just a little time.

Diaper Sign

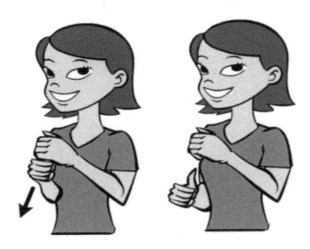

Take your hands and put them around your waist. When you're done with that, take your index and middle finger together and tap them on your thumbs.

Wet Sign

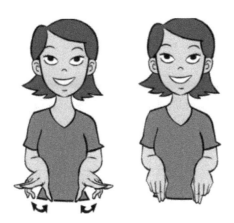

Lift your hands and bring your fingers and thumbs together and begin to pull them down. Now its sign is used when your kids want to let you know she has a wet her diaper and wants you to change it.

The Scoop On Poop

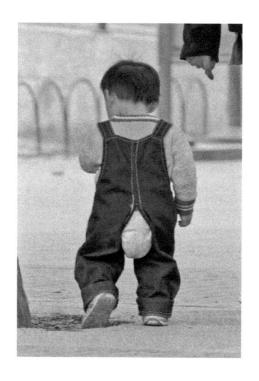

Many of the books and so-called experts on potty training tell you that your child

learns to poop in the potty long before she learns to pee. But my own unofficial

unscientific, and utterly unproven poll of real experts (a.k.a. my friends and other

actual mommies) indicates that poop training follows pee training approximately

99.9 percent of the time. (Actually, it was 100 percent, but I have to leave a little

wiggle room so I won't get sued for passing on false data.) Poop smarts can be a

far more significant challenge to learn for various reasons.

our little pooping machine indeed has an easier time recognizing the sensation of needing a bowel movement, so that part's a cinch. You may also have the added benefit of knowing when your toddler has to go poop because their bowels tend to have Swiss-timing accuracy. For these reasons, you'd think that poo training would be easy-peasy, light, and breezy. But think again. There are still plenty of hurdles to overcome when trying to get Junior to move those bowels into the potty. Going number one is a cakewalk compared with going number two. And you're like most real moms, you'll find yourself fighting for poop training long after tinkle training is achieved.

Why is it? It's anyone's guess. It could be because kids only poop once or twice a day, so they don't get the same practice time as tinkles. Issues could likewise originate from the unpredictable demonstration of cleaning that can be ignored with pee absent much exhibition. Adolescence, intense subject matters, control, dread, or outright apathy can likewise cause the crap slack. However, most likely, the main explanation behind the number-two trouble is that crap is more earnestly to manage. It smells, it spreads, it recolors—it's (a challenge I state) outright crappy.

"They," reveal to you that you shouldn't show sicken at your kid's excrement for dread that it may offend your small one. After all, the stinky poop that makes your eyes water and burns the hair in your nostrils came out of your little pride and joy. And if you respond to it negatively, "they" feel that it could send a negative message to your child and affect her self-esteem. While I understand on an intellectual level, we mommies live on a practical level, and it's tough to c in real life. Yes, you love your child unconditionally, but isn't there some loopho that says you don't have to enjoy all of her bodily functions, particularly th Olympic gold-medal winning doo-doo that just filled her diaper and leaked up t her neck?

"They" also say that boys can be much more difficult to train and take far longer t learn than girls. But why, you frantic mothers of boys might ask? Perhaps it is th emotional immaturity of boys. Probably their bowels and intestinal systems develo more slowly. Control is one of the significant issues. Because of it, some boys ca take years to train. If you're lucky, poop training won't be a huge ordeal, and he'll tak to it as naturally as he does, holding onto his penis as he falls to sleep.

Regardless of Its minor setback, let's face it—in the long run, the boys are fa more successful in the BM arena. Think of your husband, brothers, an boyfriends, even your father, any of whom could sit on the toilet and freakin poop all day! We females fight constipation from the moment we get our firs training bra and fear pooping anywhere but in the privacy of our comfortin toilets. On the other hand, males think of each "movement" like a spa day and spend long, leisurely, luxurious hours on the can getting caught up on reading.

Whether poop training comes before or after learning how to pee in the pot an whether it takes longer for boys to conquer than girls are things that only tim

. But it is going to happen at some point in the lives of your little ones. So
fore it does, let me fill you in on all the poop there is to know about, well about
op.

The Poop Hold

ou've been trying to potty-train your kid for what feels like years now. She's
en successfully making tinkle in the potty for weeks, but she has refused to take
f her diaper for the big jobs. Then, three days ago, at precisely 8:07 a.m.,
ecisely twelve minutes after she finished eating her bowl of Cap'N Crunch, the
eavens parted. She said she had to make poopie, and you marched her into the
athroom, placed her on the potty, and right on cue, she pooped! You jumped
r joy and smiled with glee. There were stickers, stars, and a small marching
and. Your mission was accomplished. You hadn't been It happy since you fit
to your pre-pregnancy jeans (okay, your pre-pregnancy fat jeans). You can now
e a happy, happy woman!

or many of you, it marks the official end of your potty-training trek. Your child
as overcome her fears and other issues in the poop department, and your job is
one. But for others—for most others—it may not be the end. It may only be
e middle. You may embark on the all-too-common "holding it in" phase, an
sue that can stay with your child for years to come. And while holding it in with
ee results in wet clothing and spots on rugs, holding it in with poop can have
ore severe consequences.

78

There are many reasons children hold onto their poop as if they were the secr

recipe for Colonel Sanders's eleven famous herbs and spices. Here are some

the most common reasons why your kid might keep his anus closed for busines

The Psychology of Poo

It seems that toddlers have two entirely different belief systems when it comes

excrement. Pee is seen as "excrement lite," and it harbors no deep-seated meanir

for toddlers. But poo can be hardcore, both figuratively and literally. (More abo

that on page 116, when we get to chat about constipation.) Toddlers attach s

much psychological significance to their poop that each dump is like its ow

Rorschach test. On some strange level, your little one sees her turd as a

extension of herself, sort of like another body part like an arm or a leg. While it

nothing to you, seeing that piece of herself flushed down the toilet can be ver

traumatic. If it is the situation you're going through, don't flush the toilet afte

she's finished. Just walk away and give it a flush as soon as you can distract he

Just don't get too distracted. If you forget to flush, your kid may come back int

the bathroom, fish it out, and use it as a source of modeling clay (more on tha

later on).

Fear Of Big Poops

can be quite scary if your little one makes a grand-, or worse, a fantasized poop. n top of it, if the stool is the least bit hard, it can most assuredly hurt. And once nappens, you'll find that you're in deep doo-doo. Now that your child associates ooping with pain, she is likely to begin holding it in. It may result in constipation d harder stools, thereby leading to even more pain and setting off the vicious cle that can spin you into insanity. If you're in the midst of its cycle, it's going take some serious support and cajoling, along with some other useful tips, to t the factory up and running again (see "Much Ado About Poo"). If It doesn't ork, call your pediatrician. He may suggest mineral oil or, in some heavy-duty ses, laxatives. Please don't try either of these solutions except on your ediatrician's advice.

Stress

1st as with grownups, stress can make children hold in their BMs. It's not necessarily conscious choice but rather has something to do with tension, causing the sphincter nuscles to constrict. Any major toddler issue like a new sibling, new babysitter, or ew sheets can cause a toddler to feel pressure, and therefore might trigger its nconscious control issue.

Traveler's Constipation

And speaking of what we big folks can relate to, how about pooping away from home? Frankly, I'm right there with the little tots on It one and find it an excellent reason to hold it in. Still, it's not the best situation to deal with—especially if your child is in daycare, at grandma's, or with you on vacation. Traveler's constipation could also become a real issue for those of you who share custody. Your child's colon may run free all week, but once she returns from a weekend at her father's she's irritable, crabby, and crammed up with crap.

Control

The most frustrating reason that a toddler controls her goods is as a conscious means of controlling you. As you know, it's easier to hold in poop than pee, and once your little dickens sets her mind to it, she can hold it in for days. It's as if she's equipped with a sphincter infused with superhero strength. All human toddlers have a special gift. They're born with it. Unfortunately, it wears off as we age, along with dewy fresh cheeks. By the time we're elderly, it may even cease to function altogether. Sad but true. It issues of control be the biggest issue that you and your child ever face—that is until your toddler becomes a teenager and wants to drop out of high school and join a band.

What generally happens is that parents, in their push to get their kids poop trained, make the massive mistake of giving the kids the message that It is mething that they want them to do. Of course, the little one then sees It as way

o much parental domination, and being the little control freak that she is,

cides to put mommy and daddy in their place.

A Brief History Of Potty Training

In the 1800s and early 1900s, children were actually potty trained at a much younger age versus today's society. Being potty trained by 18 months was not uncommon at all. It is a far cry from the statistics we get today where the average age for potty training is closer to 30 months.

Technology and family lifestyle played a significant role in pushing out the average age of potty training children. Disposable diapers didn't exist back then, and laundry machines weren't commercialized until the 1950s. Moms stayed at home to raise their kids. They had to wash soiled cloth diapers by hand unless they were rich enough to pay for a cleaning service to do the dirty work. Imagine yourself in that situation. Dirty diapers, cleaning the house, cooking the meals, mending worn clothes. It's easy to understand why women wanted to get their kids potty trained as fast as possible. It was all about eliminating diapers from their daily workload. In those times, for the husbands who went to work all day, they probably had a more straightforward job!

The potty training methods used back then were what we call "parent-centric." That is, parents potty trained their kids to reduce their workload. Parents didn't realize that forcing kids to become potty trained before they were biologically and psychologically ready could present downside risk. Enlarged ureters (the tube

...t carry urine to the outside of the body) represent a physiological risk, for ...ample.

...e first disposable diapers were invented by Marion Donovan, a New York ...usewife, during the 1950s. She was so tired of washing her kids' cloth diapers ...at she decided to cut up her shower curtains into envelope-like shapes and fill ...em with absorbent materials. She named her invention "the boater." She went ...o business selling these diapers and eventually sold the business. Today, we all ...ow that disposable diapers are a multi-billion-dollar industry.

...hile disposable diapers add convenience to our lives, they also make us lazy. ...e have accepted disposable diapers as part of the cost of raising a family. We ...ve to deal with throwing them in the trash, but it's not enough of a hassle to ...ish us to potty train our kids at a younger age, as was the case only two or three ...nerations ago.

...probably doesn't help much that most modern American families have two ...orking parents. So who has time for all It potty training stuff? It gave rise to the ...:hild-centric" potty training approach, where the parents wait for the child to be ...ady for the toilet. Child-centric training essentially translates into not pushing ...our child along to accelerate readiness.

...grew up with an engineer for a father. He taught me to think about the two ...xtremes of any situation. If either height doesn't seem right, then the better ...nswer lies somewhere in the middle. I believe potty training fits Its way of thinking entirely. The parent-centric approach is not practical and harmful to the child. The child-centric process is a result of commercialized diapers and a society where we don't mind being lazy. Neither are ideal solutions.

The process I'll teach you that accelerates potty training without ever forcing child to do anything. It's much closer to the child-centric approach than the parent-centric approach. It isn't a passive approach that encourages doing nothing. But I'll also show you how to avoid pressuring your child. It method won't result in tantrums or psychological trauma.

It saves you money, saves you time, and allow you to move onto less smelly coaching roles such as teaching your kids to swim, put on their shoes, or pour their milk.

After all, the teaching never ends. You are a coach to your child for life. Enjoy it

Constipation

Constipation in children is a severe condition that can cause potty training issue and can cause physical problems later on in life. That's why it's imperative to begin looking for constipation as soon as your child is born, but even more so during potty training exercises.

To tell if your child is constipated, look for the following signs:

Chapter 19: In newborns, firm stool that occurs less than once per day, but with difficult and straining, is constipation.

Chapter 20: Hard, dry stool and pain when passing it is constipation.

Chapter 21: A pebble-like, hard seat given by babies who strain during bowel movements, grunt, draw their legs up to the abdomen, and get red-faced constipation.

Chapter 22: Streaks of blood on the exterior of the stool is constipation.

Chapter 23: Abdominal distress, along with hard, irregular stool, is another sign of illness.

Causes

As the digested food travels through the intestines, nutrients and water are absorbed, and the waste turns into a stool. For a soft seat to be made, enough water has to stay in the waste material, and the lower rectal and intestinal muscles have to relax and contract to move the stool along and out of the body.

alfunctions of either of these mechanisms, such as not enough water or low

uscle movements, cause constipation.

ing plugged up with hard stool for three days can be uncomfortable.

onstipation can turn into a self-perpetuating issue. The hard stool causes pain

hen it passes; therefore, the child holds onto the seat. The longer the stool is

side, the harder it becomes, which makes it even more painful to pass the stool.

he muscle tone becomes weaker; the more extended the seat is in there to stretch

e intestinal wall. To complicate everything, the passage of hard stool through a

rrow rectum can tear in the rectal wall, which is known as a rectal fissure. It

eates the streaks of blood. Its painful tear make babies not want to have bowel

ovements even more.

auses of constipation in infants include:

ter 24: *New milk or foods. If your baby has begun a new meal, switched from*

rmula to breast milk or vice versa, or cow's recipe, they could be experiencing

onstipation due to its abrupt change in diet. Return to a looser-stool menu they're

sed to and slowly switch over. If you can't, then contact a pediatrician about the

roper procedure for switching.

ter 25: Causes of constipation in children include:

ter 26: Toddlers going through negative phases or emotional upsets can have a

eluctance to have a bowel movement. When people are upset, sometimes their

testines can be affected. It can cause diarrhea, too.

Chapter 27: Your toddler might not be drinking enough fluids during the day. Consid

giving them two to three extra glasses of water or some diluted juice.

Chapter 28: They might not be getting enough fiber in their diet. Consider serving mo

fresh fruits and vegetables at snack time.

<u>Treatment</u>

Try its ten-step plan to treat constipation in toddlers.

1. Serve more fluids. Not drinking enough fluids is a subtle contributor t issues when it comes to constipation, especially for young children. Th colon is the body regulator of fluids. If a person is not getting enoug fluids, their colon steals water from their waste material and gives it to the body, causing their stool to be water-deprived and hard. People who hav high-fiber diets need to increase their water consumption and fiber-ric foods because they must have water to do the intestinal cleanup job. Mor fluids in a child's diet put more liquids in their bowels, which lesse constipation.

2. Add more fiber-rich foods to their diets. Fiber softens the stool by drawin more water to them, making them easier to pass because they're bulkie Fiber foods for toddlers include graham crackers, bran cereals, whole-grai crackers and bread, and high fiber vegetables such as broccoli, peas, an beans.

3. Get them more exercise. Exercise improves digestion and speeds the passage of food through the intestines, which means less of a chance to sit and have more water sucked from it.

4. Ease the passage. Infants might need some help from their parents with some well-timed suppositories. As they go through the phase of learning how to have bowel movements, many babies in the early months draw their knees and grunt to push out their stool. However, the straining baby might appreciate some outside help with a glycerin suppository. These are available without a prescription at pharmacies and look like little rocket ships. If the baby is straining, insert one as far into the rectum as you can and hold them behind together for a few minutes to dissolve the glycerin. It helps lubricate the baby's rectum if there is a tear or bleeding. Please don't use it for more than a few days without a doctor's permission.

5. Wiggle it out. As soon as the glycerin suppository is in, wiggle it a little, which stimulates the tense muscles to relax and ease the stool's passage.

6. Insert the liquid glycerin. It is also known as Babylax, which can be inserted into the baby's rectum with a dropper and stimulate a bowel movement.

7. Use a natural laxative. When you're using a laxative, try the most natural one first. Start with diluted prune juice with the pulp. Two- to six-month-old infants should have a tablespoon or two, and toddlers should have up to eight ounces. Try strained prunes or make a puree yourself by stewing your own. You can serve it straight or disguised, or spread it on some

crackers. Apricots, plums, pears, and peaches are all laxatives, too. If the are not sufficient, then try:

a) Psyllium Husks. These are available at nutrition stores and are natural fiber sto softeners. It is a light laxative that can be served over cereal or combined with fruit and yogurt puree. Toddlers should start with one teaspoon per day an increase to two as needed. Be sure to serve it with eight ounces of water. For fiber to work, the intestines require much fluid; otherwise, the psyllium gums u and can cause worse issues.

8. Nonprescription laxatives. Malt-barley extracts and psyllium powders ca soften your child's stool, as well as these other options:

a) Flax Oil. It is a favorite for most children. It's a healthy alternative t mineral oil, which is not only a laxative but also gives your child a goo dose of omega-3 fats. While you might hear that mineral oil is good t relieve constipation, due to it being a mixture of hydrocarbons made fror petroleum products, most people are not convinced of its safety. Also unlike mineral oil, flax oil is a nutrient that helps the absorption of vitamin Infants can have up to a teaspoon a day, toddlers two, and children on tablespoon.

b) Flax Seed Meal. It is ground flaxseed, and it's a superior diuretic than the o since it has fiber in it. It seems to be like finely ground grain pieces and blend well in with soupy oats or can be added to high-fiber smoothies. The dose o

It is one tablespoon for every day for babies and two tablespoons for more seasoned youngsters.

Suppositories. Besides the glycerin suppositories alone, try suppositories that also contain a laxative ingredient. These can be used from time to time if the constipation is resistant to the more uncomplicated measures.

. Use enemas as a last resort. Babies who are constipated chronically can try something like Baby Fleet, an enema available without a prescription, and directions are on the package.

he above methods are general tips for treating or preventing constipation for all es, but they are specific to infants. It's essential to keep the bowels moving althily at an early stage because it prevents issues down the road.

Feed your infant smaller amounts of formula at more frequent intervals. It gives the intestines a good chance of adequately digesting the formula. One way to do It is to feed half as much twice as often.

Delay introducing solid foods for those who are constipated, such as bananas and rice. Rather than rice cereal, try some barley cereal. Right starter foods for infants that are high in fiber are pureed prunes and pears.

Used the glycerin suppositories to ease the passage of stools, as described above.

Add a teaspoon of flax oil into your baby's cereal or their bottle.

5. Watch out for signs they're about to go. As soon as they start to grimace, grur strain, or look bloated, quickly insert the suppository.

Bath and Bowel Movement Technique

A trick that many parents use to help ease the passage of their infant or toddle stools is to use the bath technique. It's messy, but it works. Immerse your bal in the warm bathwater, so it's surrounding them chest-high. When they're relaxe in the bathtub, massage their belly, and they'll have a bowel movement.

Iron-Fortified Formula and Constipation

Before you rush into attributing the constipation of your baby to the iron in the formul you might be interested in knowing that controlled studies performed by Dr. Oski, th Professor and Chairman of the Department of Pediatrics at John Hopkin demonstrated that iron-fortified formulas didn't cause constipation any more than method that didn't have iron.

However, scientific research and the mother's observations tend to clash. Pediatrician continue to tell you to feed your child an iron-fortified formula for a reason. Low-iro methods do not provide your baby with enough iron, resulting in anemia between th ages of six months to one year.

Toddler's Holding onto Bowel Movements

Constipation is one of the most perplexing and uncomfortable problems in young children. It is how the system is usually supposed to work—the presence of much stool in the large intestine signal the urge to go to the bathroom. The child responds to its call or chooses to ignore it if they are too busy doing something else.

Try the following steps with a toddler who is going through its cycle.

Make a diagram of their large intestine or print one out from online, showing the large golf balls of stool at the end of their large intestine. Show them that voluntarily holding it in makes them harder, and that is why it's hurting them when the stool passes.

Please encourage them to have bowel movements during the day, especially after eating breakfast.

Encourage them to respond to their urge to go immediately and convey to them that they should go when they have to go.

If your child has had its issue for a long time, the intestinal muscles can become weak. It might be necessary to try stool softeners for up to a month to correct the problem.

What Do The Experts Say?

The experts (it's the professional experts we're talking about here) agree that yc can't toilet train a child until he or she is ready physically and emotionally. Anoth is that the age of readiness varies widely from child to child.

Dr. Benjamin Spock's advice reflects the conventional wisdom. H recommendation is to use a potty chair for a child up to age two and a half rathe than a toilet seat adapter (but to use a footstool here if you do), but he admi that it's not a matter of critical importance. He recommends letting a chil become friends with the potty chair before introducing it for BMs and urinating He also adheres to the idea that the adult should not empty the potty until th child has left the room or the toilet flushed until the child loses interest in th stool before flushing, believing that for a child under two and a half, it is probabl too frightening. Let children play bottomless once a child has expressed rea interest, but if accidents occur, return to nappies. He indicates that belate backsliding on bowel control is more of a control issue, causing constipatio rather than the current theories that illness is often the culprit. Spock suggest leaving night-time training to the natural maturing of the bladder.

Dr. Brazelton's method follows a simple format. First, have your child sit (full dressed) on a potty chair at least once a day. After that ritual is accepted, undres ur child and take him or her to the potty chair. Aim for a time when your child

ikely to have a bowel movement. Praise successes, but don't overdo it. If you

l your child is ready, have your child play with no clothes on from the waist

wn, and make it clear that it is the child's responsibility to go to the potty chair

en necessary. If your child loses interest and doesn't cooperate, go back to

ppies and try again in a few weeks. Brazelton has become more accepting of

er training and has become a proponent of child-led, pressure-free toilet

ining. Emotional readiness should be the guiding factor, and pressuring a child

to be avoided. He no longer considers age four to be late for practice. His input

s part of the reason that Procter & Gamble, makers of Pampers, proceeded

th developing a more giant disposable nappy (size 6) for children over 35 lbs.

olume 6 is now familiar with the significant disposable nappy manufacturers.

r. Sears follows the basics of being sure your child is ready, that you have the

ols you need ranging from a potty seat to training pants plus patience and a

nse of humor, and teaching your child "where to go and what to call it." He

lieves in first creating a conditioned reflex that when you sit your child on the

otty, your child goes. It is best done initially by catching your child's bowel

ovement when he or she is about to go and before it is deposited in the nappy.

ake your time chart of your child's nappy bowel movements for a week or two

efore starting. With auspicious timing, a child learns its connection and

ventually makes the correct association.

John Rosemond, a family psychologist, columnist, and author, believes its proce

should be as simple and straightforward as housebreaking a puppy. He advoca

a return to traditional child-rearing practices and attributes delayed training

"wishy-washy parenting inspired by Freudian mumbo jumbo." He believes t

word "readiness" should be "capable," and kids can learn between 18 and .

months of age.

Penelope Leach discusses the fragile parity to be struck in a restroom, preparir

between guardians should be clear about their inclination for a kid to utilize t

potty or latrine yet to stay away from the impulse to use toileting as

battleground. When a kid knows about the "feeling-item" association, a youngst

ought to be informed that pee and excrement ought to be placed in a potty

latrine as adults do. She feels one should keep the impedance of a kid's day by d

exercises to a base. On the off chance that you continue reminding a youngst

to sit on the potty, you can demolish the entire cycle. Potty seats convey abili

permits it to be brought to where the youngster is so a kid can assume liability y

not need to rush to locate a potty when muscle control can't practice that sort

postponement. Keeping away from nappies is suggested, and be ready fc

puddles. Praise with joy, yet don't go over the edge with congrats.

Louise Bates Ames of the Gessell Institute of Child Development considers eac

to be a quieter about its formative assignment than its ancestor. She, despit

everything, suggests utilizing the paper on-the-restroom floor routine for a ki

…d generally a kid) who demands hunching down for a BM and not use either …otty seat or the latrine until It stage passes.

…former bestselling toilet training book that has made enthusiastic converts of …me and sparked controversy among others is Toilet Training in Less Than a …ay by Nathan Azrin, Ph.D., and Richard Foxx, Ph.D. The program these two …ychologists recommend was first devised not for speed, but to help the mentally …sabled learn its difficult skill. Later, it was adapted for the average child. Some …ople feel that the program is overly manipulative and, in some aspects, actually …nitive. Others object to the heavy use of sweet drinks, sweets, and salty treats.

The Demands Of Both Parent And Child Are Considerable.

…ne whole day must be devoted to training, with no distractions whatsoever. The …athors recommend that trainers and trainees be confined to the kitchen, where …ean-up is comparatively easy. Here's a summary of the procedure:

1. The parent provides a doll that wets and, with prompting from the parent, the child "trains" the baby in the prescribed manner.

2. Liquids are continuously offered, on the theory that the more urine produced, the more quickly the training be accomplished. Salty snacks are given freely, if necessary, to increase appetite for the liquids.

3. The parent is given a sequence of reminders to use, ranging from a firm "go now" to questions about the need to go and general suggestions.

4. The child goes to the potty, pulls down his or her pants (very loose ones are recommended), and sits there for ten minutes, or until urination occurs. The child wipes himself or herself and pulls up the pants.

5. Four rewards are given for every success: verbal praise, nonverbal reinforcement (hugs and kisses), something good to eat, and reference to "friends who care" ("Grandma be so pleased"; "Tommy goes in the potty, too").

6. Disapproval is expressed when there's an accident, although ". . . spanking or other physical punishment is probably never justified." The child is then required to practice hurrying to the potty from different places in the house ten times (yes, 10!), to feel the pants to tell the difference between wet and dry, and finally, to do all the necessary clean up.

But does it work? Many say it does. And in a formal study of children 20 months to four-plus years of age, Azrin and Foxx found that success was achieved in periods ranging from a half-hour to two days, with the average being about four hours.

sponses to a question about the method varied:

oilet Training in Less Than a Day was our biggest help. (My son was two years, ne months.) The two disadvantages were 1) it was very boring for me, and 2) u should stay home for a week to be sure the method has stuck. Very much orth it."

ancy Holte

Jnless your child is eager to please you in general, the boundaries are so rigid at you may have a major battle."

laine Whitlock

have concluded that when your child is ready, he'll do it. I used TTLD for my first n when he was about three years old, and it worked! It was beautiful, and I told eryone about that book-until I tried with son number two, and it failed miserably! ow, seven months later, he's trained, and to its day, I still don't know what caused it happen other than that he was ready, that all the explaining, practicing-not to mention ie big-boy pants with the trucks on them-finally clicked, and he understood.

Using Rewards

oilet training in less than a day emphasizes the reward system, which has raised gnificant concern for parents. Many parents feel strongly that any kind of iaterial reward is wrong or merely inappropriate when a child is learning necessary, proper behavior. Others don't object at all. And some objects only the use of sweets. Don't think of this as bribery. This is behavior modification.

The biggest concern of those offering rewards is, "How and when do I stop "Will, my child, expect a treat or gift every time he or she visits the bathroom f weeks, months, or years?"

According to parents who have used the reward system, this is not a problem. is easy to run out of whatever you are using after a few weeks. Kids do accep that. And a reward system can be an effective motivator!

You can differentiate rewards as you progress. When your child either asks to go witho prompting (and makes it to the potty on time) or spontaneously uses the pot independently or attains a certain number of dry days, it might be the time for a "large reward that has been known before.

Our son would willingly pee in the toilet or potty, but a bowel movement h would only do in his pants. My husband came up with the ideas of "pennies fc poos," which worked for us. It was better than sweets and boosted his ban balance. We now have a six-month-old girl, and we've already started savin change!

Mary Jackson

Use your imagination for rewards (you know your child best), and conside combining material rewards with nonmaterial ones. For some children, the mos ful tip might be calling grandpa or grandma to report a "success" (this works

st if grandparents live within local dialing distance!); for others, it's stickers or

rs on a chart, calendar, or even the potty itself. Letting your child pick out

orite stickers at a store can add to their interest. One child I know was

tivated by the promise of wearing a swimsuit all day long if there were no

idents, while a set number of pushes on a swing did the trick for another child.

cement of any tangible rewards to be handed out is helpful too. They should

in sight but out of reach. A large, clear canister or bowl is one way to

complish this. Or they are maybe having an assortment of small wrapped items

red in the bathroom.

CONCLUSION

Thank you for reading all this book!

Sense of Self

A Montessori class consists of students with typically three years of age. Ideal students and teachers stick with the course, build a supportive environment, an positive relationships during the period.

Students of different ages are commonly seen to work together. Older student love mentoring their younger peers – someone who has recently learned the tas at hand is often the better instructor. Younger students gaze at their big brother and sisters and have an idea of the enticing work to be done.

As children mature over the three years in the Montessori classroom, they realiz that they belong to a community where each one has his / her individual need but also the neighborhood. Kids are free but still have the opportunity t collaborate with their friends and support them while they are in need.

To achieve independence and self-interest in a caring community, every studer has a strong sense of self and encourages pride in their individuality.

ch child has the chance to progress at its speed and developmental stage. erything about a Montessori classroom is well designed to support the child's merging independence from an early age and is usually known as 'prepared vironments.' As each year progresses, all children have opportunities to velop more responsibility, freedom, positive decisions, and active learning.

ie Italian pediatrician and pioneering educator who began the technique, Dr. aria Montessori, claimed that a self-confiding, interested, and the imaginative iild develops in children who can select their own learning experiences. As it rns out, the parents are looking for this approach, which is 100 years old.

ontessori's main objective is to provide children with a stimulating environment which they can explore, touch, and learn without fear. In its own pace, every iild learns. Teachers understand and inspire children to love learning and to feel od with their experience and meaning in life. Here are some of the advantages:

hools in Montessori teach early independence. Children are actively involved running their school, such as preparing and serving drinks and using learning juipment. Practically, the kids learn new things every day, such as sweeping, olishing, making snacks, and tying shoelaces.

ontrary to the method of conventional schools, children are not expected to omply with set standards of success. The Montessori procedure takes into onsideration every child's needs, talents, gifts, and particular personalities. The children learn at their own pace, so what they do is not restricted or criticize. There is complete freedom to comprehend, which makes it fun to learn.

Each child optimizes their full potential, irrespective of their ability or interest. All kids fit in, including kids with learning handicaps. Many kids learn best, and the equipment has been designed for this. For instance, the sand alphabet – sand letters on the card – is one piece of equipment. The child with his finger follows the sand letter and then writes the letter on paper. There are things of interest to the child for all subjects, but he learns best. For example, not only books but globes, mapping puzzles, images, and pictures of animals (sensorial items) are present in geography.

Regular visits are also made to people, animals, pets, and various activities depending on the subject, for example—Chinese cuisine, sampling Italian food, etc.

Children are encouraged to respect and assist one another in a Montessori environment. If you choose, you are working with other kids and helping each other or 'teaching. Watching kids who want to help each other is lovely.

You have already taken a step towards your improvement.
Best wishes!

CPSIA information can be obtained
at www.ICGtesting.com
Printed in the USA
BVHW082317030521
606340BV00007B/1669